T0199910

# SCHIZOPHRENIA
## SPECTRUM AND OTHER PSYCHOTIC
# DISORDERS

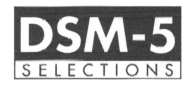

# SCHIZOPHRENIA
## SPECTRUM AND OTHER PSYCHOTIC
# DISORDERS

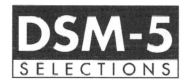

## American Psychiatric Association

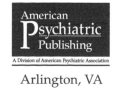

American Psychiatric Publishing
A Division of American Psychiatric Association

Arlington, VA

Copyright © 2016 American Psychiatric Association

DSM® and DSM-5® are registered trademarks of the American Psychiatric Association. Use of these terms is prohibited without permission of the American Psychiatric Association.

ALL RIGHTS RESERVED. Unless authorized in writing by the APA, no part of this book may be reproduced or used in a manner inconsistent with the APA's copyright. This prohibition applies to unauthorized uses or reproductions in any form, including electronic applications.

Correspondence regarding copyright permissions should be directed to Permissions, American Psychiatric Publishing, 1000 Wilson Boulevard, Suite 1825, Arlington, VA 22209-3901.

Manufactured in the United States of America on acid-free paper.

ISBN 978-1-61537-011-5 (Paperback)

American Psychiatric Association
1000 Wilson Boulevard
Arlington, VA 22209-3901
www.psych.org

*Schizophrenia Spectrum and Other Psychotic Disorders: DSM-5® Selections* is an anthology published by the American Psychiatric Association from the following sources:

American Psychiatric Association: *Diagnostic and Statistical Manual of Mental Disorders*, Fifth Edition. Arlington, VA, American Psychiatric Association, 2013

Black DW, Grant JE: *DSM-5® Guidebook: The Essential Companion to the Diagnostic and Statistical Manual of Mental Disorders, Fifth Edition.* Washington, DC, American Psychiatric Publishing, 2014

Barnhill JW: *DSM-5® Clinical Cases.* Washington, DC, American Psychiatric Publishing, 2014

Muskin PR: *DSM-5® Self-Exam Questions: Test Questions for the Diagnostic Criteria.* Washington, DC, American Psychiatric Publishing, 2014

# Contents

# Introduction to DSM-5® Selections

Welcome to *DSM-5 Selections*. The purpose of this series is to educate readers about important diagnostic issues associated with categories of DSM-5 disorders. The initial books in the *DSM-5 Selections* series are *Sleep-Wake Disorders, Depressive Disorders, Schizophrenia Spectrum and Other Psychotic Disorders, Feeding and Eating Disorders, Neurodevelopmental Disorders*, and *Anxiety Disorders*. Each book in the series includes the diagnostic criteria relevant to the disorders included in each category. The criteria are taken directly from DSM-5, the most comprehensive, current, and critical resource for clinical practice available today. Also included in each book in the series are extracts from the *DSM-5 Guidebook, DSM-5 Clinical Cases,* and *DSM-5 Self-Exam Questions.* Consequently, each book in the series offers readers a unique introduction to individual categories of DSM-5 disorders and an opportunity to test one's knowledge about DSM-5 disorders.

*DSM-5 Guidebook* serves as a roadmap to DSM-5 disorders for clinicians and researchers. It illuminates the content of DSM-5 by teaching mental health professionals how to use the revised diagnostic criteria, and it provides practical content for its clinical use. The book offers a fresh perspective to DSM diagnostic categories by focusing on the changes between DSM-IV-TR and DSM-5 that will most significantly impact clinical application of the criteria.

*DSM-5 Clinical Cases* presents composite patient cases that exemplify the diagnostic criteria for disorders contained in a category. *DSM-5 Clinical Cases* makes DSM-5 come alive for teachers, students, and clinicians. The book helps readers to understand diagnostic concepts, including symptoms, severity, comorbidities, age of onset and development, dimensionality across disorders, and gender and cultural implications.

The questions in *DSM-5 Self-Exam Questions* were written to test readers' knowledge of conceptual changes to DSM-5, specific changes to diagnoses, and the diagnostic criteria. Each question includes short answers that explain the rationale for each correct answer and contain important information on diagnostic classification, criteria sets, diagnoses, codes, severity, culture, age, and gender. The questions are helpful for preparing for various examinations.

The *DSM-5 Selections* series is not intended to replace DSM-5 or the other books from which the extracts are taken. Rather, the series is intended to give readers key selected materials that pertain directly to specific disorder categories. If you find that you require more information about a specific disorder or category of disorders, you are encouraged to examine an APP textbook or clinical manual. You can review the full list of APP titles at www.appi.org.

Robert E. Hales, M.D.
Editor-in-Chief

# Preface

There are 12 mental disorders in the "Schizophrenia Spectrum and Other Psychotic Disorders" chapter of DSM-5. In addition to schizophrenia, the disorders in this section include schizophreniform disorder, brief psychotic disorder, schizoaffective disorder, delusional disorder, schizotypal (personality) disorder, and catatonia. Like other disorders in DSM-5, schizophrenia and psychotic disorders can be drug- or medication-induced or due to another medical condition.

Schizophrenia is a brain disorder that affects how people think, feel, and behave. The course of the illness is quite variable, and outcomes range from complete recovery to severe disability. As you will see from reading the material contained in this book, the most prominent characteristics of schizophrenia are hallucinations, delusions, and disorganized thinking. In addition, patients with this disorder exhibit negative symptoms, which are more difficult to recognize. Examples of negative symptoms include social withdrawal and diminished emotional engagement.

The usual age at onset of schizophrenia is during late adolescence or early adulthood. As a result, schizophrenia and other psychotic disorders can be leading causes of disability during a patient's lifetime. For example, throughout the world, schizophrenia is a leading cause of disability for both men and women. Examples of disability include unemployment, violence, hospitalizations, medical illnesses, homelessness, and premature mortality.

Worldwide, the prevalence of schizophrenia is estimated to be 1%, but it may be higher. There are significant variations in this illness across populations. Unfortunately, many individuals with schizophrenia do not receive the treatment that they need.

The course of schizophrenia ranges from complete recovery to chronicity. Usually, patients who experience a first episode of psychosis will experience remission, but almost all will relapse at some time. Approximately 20% of individuals who develop a schizophrenic disorder will have sustained recovery, and a small proportion of these will completely recover and never relapse. Although approximately one-third of patients achieve a relatively good outcome, the remaining two-thirds will have moderate to severe symptoms and functional impairments. Approximately 10% of patients will have persistent and unremitting psychosis. Clinicians often have a pessimistic view of this disorder because they only see patients with persistent or recurrent symptoms and significant functional disability. They rarely see patients who recover and never relapse.

Schizophrenia spectrum and other psychotic disorders are important disorders to diagnose, understand, and treat. Early diagnosis and treatment can change the trajec-

---

Adapted with permission from Stroup TS, Lawrence RE, Abbas AI, et al.: "Schizophrenia Spectrum and Other Psychotic Disorders," in *The American Psychiatric Publishing Textbook of Psychiatry*, 6th Edition. Edited by Hales RE, Yudofsky SC, Roberts LW. Washington, DC, American Psychiatric Publishing, 2014, pp. 273–309.

tory of a person's life. The material contained in this book will help clinicians to better understand and diagnose patients suffering from a schizophrenia spectrum disorder.

# Highlights of Changes From DSM-IV-TR to DSM-5

Two changes were made to DSM-IV Criterion A for schizophrenia. The first change is the elimination of the special attribution of bizarre delusions and Schneiderian first-rank auditory hallucinations (e.g., two or more voices conversing). In DSM-IV, only one such symptom was needed to meet the diagnostic requirement for Criterion A, instead of two of the other listed symptoms. This special attribution was removed because of the nonspecificity of Schneiderian symptoms and the poor reliability in distinguishing bizarre from nonbizarre delusions. Therefore, in DSM-5, two Criterion A symptoms are required for any diagnosis of schizophrenia. The second change is the addition of a requirement in Criterion A that the individual must have at least one of these three symptoms: delusions, hallucinations, and disorganized speech. At least one of these core "positive symptoms" is necessary for a reliable diagnosis of schizophrenia.

## Schizophrenia Subtypes

The DSM-IV subtypes of schizophrenia (i.e., paranoid, disorganized, catatonic, undifferentiated, and residual types) were eliminated because of their limited diagnostic stability, low reliability, and poor validity. These subtypes also have not been shown to exhibit distinctive patterns of treatment response or longitudinal course. Instead, a dimensional approach to rating severity for the core symptoms of schizophrenia is included in DSM-5 Section III to capture the important heterogeneity in symptom type and severity expressed across individuals with psychotic disorders.

## Schizoaffective Disorder

The primary change to schizoaffective disorder is the requirement that a major mood episode be present for a majority of the disorder's total duration after Criterion A has been met. This change was made on both conceptual and psychometric grounds. It makes schizoaffective disorder a longitudinal instead of a cross-sectional diagnosis—more comparable to schizophrenia, bipolar disorder, and major depressive disorder, which are bridged by this condition. The change was also made to improve the reliability, diagnostic stability, and validity of this disorder, while recognizing that the characterization of patients with both psychotic and mood symptoms, either concurrently or at different points in their illness, has been a clinical challenge.

## Delusional Disorder

Criterion A for delusional disorder no longer has the requirement that the delusions must be nonbizarre. A specifier for bizarre delusions ("with bizarre content") provides continuity with DSM-IV. The demarcation of delusional disorder from psychotic variants of obsessive-compulsive disorder and body dysmorphic disorder is explicitly noted with a new exclusion criterion, which states that the symptoms must not be better explained by conditions such as obsessive-compulsive or body dysmorphic disorder with absent insight/delusional beliefs. DSM-5 no longer separates delusional disorder from shared delusional disorder. If criteria are met for delusional disorder, then that diagnosis is made. If the diagnosis cannot be made but shared beliefs are present, then the diagnosis *other specified schizophrenia spectrum and other psychotic disorder* is used.

## Catatonia

The same criteria are used to diagnose catatonia whether the context is a psychotic, bipolar, depressive, or other medical disorder or an unidentified medical condition. In DSM-IV, two out of five symptom clusters were required if the context was a psychotic or mood disorder, whereas only one symptom cluster was needed if the context was a general medical condition. In DSM-5, all contexts require three catatonic symptoms (from a total of 12 characteristic symptoms). In DSM-5, catatonia may be diagnosed as a specifier for depressive, bipolar, and psychotic disorders; as a separate diagnosis in the context of another medical condition; or as an other specified diagnosis.

# DSM-5® Schizophrenia Spectrum and Other Psychotic Disorders: ICD-9-CM and ICD-10-CM Codes

| Disorder | ICD-9-CM | ICD-10-CM |
|---|---|---|
| Schizotypal (Personality) Disorder | 301.22 | F21 |
| Delusional Disorder | 297.1 | F22 |
| Brief Psychotic Disorder | 298.8 | F23 |
| Schizophreniform Disorder | 295.40 | F20.81 |
| Schizophrenia | 295.90 | F20.9 |
| Schizoaffective Disorder | | |
|     Bipolar type | 295.70 | F25.0 |
|     Depressive type | 295.70 | F25.1 |
| Substance/Medication-Induced Psychotic Disorder | See table below | |
| Psychotic Disorder Due to Another Condition | | |
|     With delusions | 293.81 | F06.2 |
|     With hallucinations | 293.82 | F06.0 |
| Catatonia | | |
|     Catatonia Associated With Another Mental Disorder (Catatonia Specifier) | 293.89 | F06.1 |
|     Catatonic Disorder Due to Another Medical Condition | 293.89 | F06.1 |
|     Unspecified Catatonia | 293.89 | F06.1 |
| Other Specified Schizophrenia Spectrum and Other Psychotic Disorder | 298.8 | F28 |
| Unspecified Schizophrenia Spectrum and Other Psychotic Disorder | 298.9 | F29 |

## Substance/Medication-Induced Psychotic Disorder

| | ICD-9-CM | ICD-10-CM | | |
| --- | --- | --- | --- | --- |
| | | With use disorder, mild | With use disorder, moderate or severe | Without use disorder |
| Alcohol | 291.9 | F10.159 | F10.259 | F10.959 |
| Cannabis | 292.9 | F12.159 | F12.259 | F12.959 |
| Phencyclidine | 292.9 | F16.159 | F16.259 | F16.959 |
| Other hallucinogen | 292.9 | F16.159 | F16.259 | F16.959 |
| Inhalant | 292.9 | F18.159 | F18.259 | F18.959 |
| Sedative, hypnotic, or anxiolytic | 292.9 | F13.159 | F13.259 | F13.959 |
| Amphetamine (or other stimulant) | 292.9 | F15.159 | F15.259 | F15.959 |
| Cocaine | 292.9 | F14.159 | F14.259 | F14.959 |
| Other (or unknown) substance | 292.9 | F19.159 | F19.259 | F19.959 |

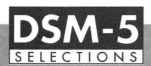

# Schizophrenia Spectrum and Other Psychotic Disorders
## Diagnostic and Statistical Manual of Mental Disorders, Fifth Edition

Schizophrenia spectrum and other psychotic disorders include schizophrenia, other psychotic disorders, and schizotypal (personality) disorder. They are defined by abnormalities in one or more of the following five domains: delusions, hallucinations, disorganized thinking (speech), grossly disorganized or abnormal motor behavior (including catatonia), and negative symptoms.

# Key Features That Define the Psychotic Disorders

## Delusions

*Delusions* are fixed beliefs that are not amenable to change in light of conflicting evidence. Their content may include a variety of themes (e.g., persecutory, referential, somatic, religious, grandiose). *Persecutory delusions* (i.e., belief that one is going to be harmed, harassed, and so forth by an individual, organization, or other group) are most common. *Referential delusions* (i.e., belief that certain gestures, comments, environmental cues, and so forth are directed at oneself) are also common. *Grandiose delusions* (i.e., when an individual believes that he or she has exceptional abilities, wealth, or fame) and *erotomanic delusions* (i.e., when an individual believes falsely that another person is in love with him or her) are also seen. *Nihilistic delusions* involve the conviction that a major catastrophe will occur, and *somatic delusions* focus on preoccupations regarding health and organ function.

Delusions are deemed *bizarre* if they are clearly implausible and not understandable to same-culture peers and do not derive from ordinary life experiences. An example of a bizarre delusion is the belief that an outside force has removed his or her internal organs and replaced them with someone else's organs without leaving any wounds or scars. An example of a nonbizarre delusion is the belief that one is under surveillance by the police, despite a lack of convincing evidence. Delusions that express a loss of control over mind or body are generally considered to be bizarre; these include the belief that one's thoughts have been "removed" by some outside force (*thought withdrawal*), that alien thoughts have been put into one's mind (*thought insertion*), or that one's body or actions are being acted on or manipulated by some outside force (*delusions of control*). The

1

distinction between a delusion and a strongly held idea is sometimes difficult to make and depends in part on the degree of conviction with which the belief is held despite clear or reasonable contradictory evidence regarding its veracity.

## Hallucinations

*Hallucinations* are perception-like experiences that occur without an external stimulus. They are vivid and clear, with the full force and impact of normal perceptions, and not under voluntary control. They may occur in any sensory modality, but auditory hallucinations are the most common in schizophrenia and related disorders. Auditory hallucinations are usually experienced as voices, whether familiar or unfamiliar, that are perceived as distinct from the individual's own thoughts. The hallucinations must occur in the context of a clear sensorium; those that occur while falling asleep (*hypnagogic*) or waking up (*hypnopompic*) are considered to be within the range of normal experience. Hallucinations may be a normal part of religious experience in certain cultural contexts.

## Disorganized Thinking (Speech)

*Disorganized thinking* (*formal thought disorder*) is typically inferred from the individual's speech. The individual may switch from one topic to another (*derailment or loose associations*). Answers to questions may be obliquely related or completely unrelated (*tangentiality*). Rarely, speech may be so severely disorganized that it is nearly incomprehensible and resembles receptive aphasia in its linguistic disorganization (*incoherence* or "word salad"). Because mildly disorganized speech is common and nonspecific, the symptom must be severe enough to substantially impair effective communication. The severity of the impairment may be difficult to evaluate if the person making the diagnosis comes from a different linguistic background than that of the person being examined. Less severe disorganized thinking or speech may occur during the prodromal and residual periods of schizophrenia.

## Grossly Disorganized or Abnormal Motor Behavior (Including Catatonia)

*Grossly disorganized or abnormal motor behavior* may manifest itself in a variety of ways, ranging from childlike "silliness" to unpredictable agitation. Problems may be noted in any form of goal-directed behavior, leading to difficulties in performing activities of daily living.

*Catatonic behavior* is a marked decrease in reactivity to the environment. This ranges from resistance to instructions (*negativism*); to maintaining a rigid, inappropriate or bizarre posture; to a complete lack of verbal and motor responses (*mutism* and *stupor*). It can also include purposeless and excessive motor activity without obvious cause (*catatonic excitement*). Other features are repeated stereotyped movements, staring, grimacing, mutism, and the echoing of speech. Although catatonia has historically been associated with schizophrenia, catatonic symptoms are nonspecific and may occur in other mental disorders (e.g., bipolar or depressive disorders with catatonia) and in medical conditions (catatonic disorder due to another medical condition).

## Negative Symptoms

*Negative symptoms* account for a substantial portion of the morbidity associated with schizophrenia but are less prominent in other psychotic disorders. Two negative symptoms are particularly prominent in schizophrenia: diminished emotional expression and avolition. *Diminished emotional expression* includes reductions in the expression of emotions in the face, eye contact, intonation of speech (prosody), and movements of the hand, head, and face that normally give an emotional emphasis to speech. *Avolition* is a decrease in motivated self-initiated purposeful activities. The individual may sit for long periods of time and show little interest in participating in work or social activities. Other negative symptoms include alogia, anhedonia, and asociality. *Alogia* is manifested by diminished speech output. *Anhedonia* is the decreased ability to experience pleasure from positive stimuli or a degradation in the recollection of pleasure previously experienced. *Asociality* refers to the apparent lack of interest in social interactions and may be associated with avolition, but it can also be a manifestation of limited opportunities for social interactions.

# Disorders in This Chapter

This chapter is organized along a gradient of psychopathology. Clinicians should first consider conditions that do not reach full criteria for a psychotic disorder or are limited to one domain of psychopathology. Then they should consider time-limited conditions. Finally, the diagnosis of a schizophrenia spectrum disorder requires the exclusion of another condition that may give rise to psychosis.

Schizotypal personality disorder is noted within this chapter as it is considered within the schizophrenia spectrum, although its full description is found in the DSM-5 chapter "Personality Disorders." The diagnosis schizotypal personality disorder captures a pervasive pattern of social and interpersonal deficits, including reduced capacity for close relationships; cognitive or perceptual distortions; and eccentricities of behavior, usually beginning by early adulthood but in some cases first becoming apparent in childhood and adolescence. Abnormalities of beliefs, thinking, and perception are below the threshold for the diagnosis of a psychotic disorder.

Two conditions are defined by abnormalities limited to one domain of psychosis: delusions or catatonia. Delusional disorder is characterized by at least 1 month of delusions but no other psychotic symptoms. Catatonia is described later in the chapter and further in this discussion.

Brief psychotic disorder lasts more than 1 day and remits by 1 month. Schizophreniform disorder is characterized by a symptomatic presentation equivalent to that of schizophrenia except for its duration (less than 6 months) and the absence of a requirement for a decline in functioning.

Schizophrenia lasts for at least 6 months and includes at least 1 month of active-phase symptoms. In schizoaffective disorder, a mood episode and the active-phase symptoms of schizophrenia occur together and were preceded or are followed by at least 2 weeks of delusions or hallucinations without prominent mood symptoms.

Psychotic disorders may be induced by another condition. In substance/medication-induced psychotic disorder, the psychotic symptoms are judged to be a physiological consequence of a drug of abuse, a medication, or toxin exposure and cease after removal of the agent. In psychotic disorder due to another medical condition, the psychotic symptoms are judged to be a direct physiological consequence of another medical condition.

Catatonia can occur in several disorders, including neurodevelopmental, psychotic, bipolar, depressive, and other mental disorders. This chapter also includes the diagnoses catatonia associated with another mental disorder (catatonia specifier), catatonic disorder due to another medical condition, and unspecified catatonia, and the diagnostic criteria for all three conditions are described together.

Other specified and unspecified schizophrenia spectrum and other psychotic disorders are included for classifying psychotic presentations that do not meet the criteria for any of the specific psychotic disorders or psychotic symptomatology about which there is inadequate or contradictory information.

# Clinician-Rated Assessment of Symptoms and Related Clinical Phenomena in Psychosis

Psychotic disorders are heterogeneous, and the severity of symptoms can predict important aspects of the illness, such as the degree of cognitive or neurobiological deficits. To move the field forward, a detailed framework for the assessment of severity is included in DSM-5 Section III "Assessment Measures," which may help with treatment planning, prognostic decision making, and research on pathophysiological mechanisms. Section III "Assessment Measures" also contains dimensional assessments of the primary symptoms of psychosis, including hallucinations, delusions, disorganized speech (except for substance/medication-induced psychotic disorder and psychotic disorder due to another medical condition), abnormal psychomotor behavior, and negative symptoms, as well as dimensional assessments of depression and mania. The severity of mood symptoms in psychosis has prognostic value and guides treatment. There is growing evidence that schizoaffective disorder is not a distinct nosological category. Thus, dimensional assessments of depression and mania for all psychotic disorders alert clinicians to mood pathology and the need to treat where appropriate. The Section III scale also includes a dimensional assessment of cognitive impairment. Many individuals with psychotic disorders have impairments in a range of cognitive domains that predict functional status. Clinical neuropsychological assessment can help guide diagnosis and treatment, but brief assessments without formal neuropsychological assessment can provide useful information that can be sufficient for diagnostic purposes. Formal neuropsychological testing, when conducted, should be administered and scored by personnel trained in the use of testing instruments. If a formal neuropsychological assessment is not conducted, the clinician should use the best available information to make a judgment. Further research on these assessments is necessary in order to determine their clinical utility; thus, the assessments available in Section III should serve as a prototype to stimulate such research.

# Schizotypal (Personality) Disorder

Criteria and text for schizotypal personality disorder can be found in the DSM-5 chapter "Personality Disorders." Because this disorder is considered part of the schizophrenia spectrum of disorders, and is labeled in this section of ICD-9 and ICD-10 as schizotypal disorder, it is listed in this chapter and discussed in detail in the DSM-5 chapter "Personality Disorders."

# Delusional Disorder

## Diagnostic Criteria                                                297.1 (F22)

A. The presence of one (or more) delusions with a duration of 1 month or longer.

B. Criterion A for schizophrenia has never been met.

   **Note:** Hallucinations, if present, are not prominent and are related to the delusional theme (e.g., the sensation of being infested with insects associated with delusions of infestation).

C. Apart from the impact of the delusion(s) or its ramifications, functioning is not markedly impaired, and behavior is not obviously bizarre or odd.

D. If manic or major depressive episodes have occurred, these have been brief relative to the duration of the delusional periods.

E. The disturbance is not attributable to the physiological effects of a substance or another medical condition and is not better explained by another mental disorder, such as body dysmorphic disorder or obsessive-compulsive disorder.

*Specify* whether:

   **Erotomanic type:** This subtype applies when the central theme of the delusion is that another person is in love with the individual.

   **Grandiose type:** This subtype applies when the central theme of the delusion is the conviction of having some great (but unrecognized) talent or insight or having made some important discovery.

   **Jealous type:** This subtype applies when the central theme of the individual's delusion is that his or her spouse or lover is unfaithful.

   **Persecutory type:** This subtype applies when the central theme of the delusion involves the individual's belief that he or she is being conspired against, cheated, spied on, followed, poisoned or drugged, maliciously maligned, harassed, or obstructed in the pursuit of long-term goals.

   **Somatic type:** This subtype applies when the central theme of the delusion involves bodily functions or sensations.

   **Mixed type:** This subtype applies when no one delusional theme predominates.

   **Unspecified type:** This subtype applies when the dominant delusional belief cannot be clearly determined or is not described in the specific types (e.g., referential delusions without a prominent persecutory or grandiose component).

*Specify* if:

   **With bizarre content:** Delusions are deemed bizarre if they are clearly implausible, not understandable, and not derived from ordinary life experiences (e.g., an individual's belief that a stranger has removed his or her internal organs and replaced them with someone else's organs without leaving any wounds or scars).

*Specify* if:

The following course specifiers are only to be used after a 1-year duration of the disorder:

**First episode, currently in acute episode:** First manifestation of the disorder meeting the defining diagnostic symptom and time criteria. An *acute episode* is a time period in which the symptom criteria are fulfilled.

**First episode, currently in partial remission:** *Partial remission* is a time period during which an improvement after a previous episode is maintained and in which the defining criteria of the disorder are only partially fulfilled.

**First episode, currently in full remission:** *Full remission* is a period of time after a previous episode during which no disorder-specific symptoms are present.

**Multiple episodes, currently in acute episode**

**Multiple episodes, currently in partial remission**

**Multiple episodes, currently in full remission**

**Continuous:** Symptoms fulfilling the diagnostic symptom criteria of the disorder are remaining for the majority of the illness course, with subthreshold symptom periods being very brief relative to the overall course.

**Unspecified**

*Specify* current severity:

Severity is rated by a quantitative assessment of the primary symptoms of psychosis, including delusions, hallucinations, disorganized speech, abnormal psychomotor behavior, and negative symptoms. Each of these symptoms may be rated for its current severity (most severe in the last 7 days) on a 5-point scale ranging from 0 (not present) to 4 (present and severe). (See Clinician-Rated Dimensions of Psychosis Symptom Severity in the chapter "Assessment Measures" [in DSM-5].)

**Note:** Diagnosis of delusional disorder can be made without using this severity specifier.

## Subtypes

In *erotomanic type,* the central theme of the delusion is that another person is in love with the individual. The person about whom this conviction is held is usually of higher status (e.g., a famous individual or a superior at work) but can be a complete stranger. Efforts to contact the object of the delusion are common. In *grandiose type,* the central theme of the delusion is the conviction of having some great talent or insight or of having made some important discovery. Less commonly, the individual may have the delusion of having a special relationship with a prominent individual or of being a prominent person (in which case the actual individual may be regarded as an impostor). Grandiose delusions may have a religious content. In *jealous type,* the central theme of the delusion is that of an unfaithful partner. This belief is arrived at without due cause and is based on incorrect inferences supported by small bits of "evidence" (e.g., disarrayed clothing). The individual with the delusion usually confronts the spouse or lover and attempts to intervene in the imagined infidelity. In *persecutory type,* the central theme of the delusion involves the individual's belief of being conspired against, cheated, spied on, followed, poisoned, maliciously maligned, harassed, or obstructed in the pursuit of long-term goals. Small slights may be exaggerated and become the focus of a delusional system. The affected individual may engage in repeated attempts to obtain satisfaction by legal or legislative action. Individuals with persecutory delusions are often resentful and angry and may resort to violence against those they believe are hurting them. In *somatic type,* the central theme of the delusion involves bodily functions or sensations. Somatic delusions can occur in several forms. Most common is the belief that the individual emits a foul odor; that there is an infestation of insects on or in the skin; that there is an internal parasite; that certain parts of the body are misshapen or ugly; or that parts of the body are not functioning.

## Diagnostic Features

The essential feature of delusional disorder is the presence of one or more delusions that persist for at least 1 month (Criterion A). A diagnosis of delusional disorder is not given if the individual has ever had a symptom presentation that met Criterion A for schizophrenia (Criterion B). Apart from the direct impact of the delusions, impairments in psychosocial functioning may be more circumscribed than those seen in other psychotic disorders such as schizophrenia, and behavior is not obviously bizarre or odd (Criterion C). If mood episodes occur concurrently with the delusions, the total duration of these mood episodes is brief relative to the total duration of the delusional periods (Criterion D). The delusions are not attributable to the physiological effects of a substance (e.g., cocaine) or another medical condition (e.g., Alzheimer's disease) and are not better explained by another mental disorder, such as body dysmorphic disorder or obsessive-compulsive disorder (Criterion E).

In addition to the five symptom domain areas identified in the diagnostic criteria, the assessment of cognition, depression, and mania symptom domains is vital for making critically important distinctions between the various schizophrenia spectrum and other psychotic disorders.

## Associated Features Supporting Diagnosis

Social, marital, or work problems can result from the delusional beliefs of delusional disorder. Individuals with delusional disorder may be able to factually describe that others view their beliefs as irrational but are unable to accept this themselves (i.e., there may be "factual insight" but no true insight). Many individuals develop irritable or dysphoric mood, which can usually be understood as a reaction to their delusional beliefs. Anger and violent behavior can occur with persecutory, jealous, and erotomanic types. The individual may engage in litigious or antagonistic behavior (e.g., sending hundreds of letters of protest to the government). Legal difficulties can occur, particularly in jealous and erotomanic types.

## Prevalence

The lifetime prevalence of delusional disorder has been estimated at around 0.2%, and the most frequent subtype is persecutory. Delusional disorder, jealous type, is probably more common in males than in females, but there are no major gender differences in the overall frequency of delusional disorder.

## Development and Course

On average, global function is generally better than that observed in schizophrenia. Although the diagnosis is generally stable, a proportion of individuals go on to develop schizophrenia. Delusional disorder has a significant familial relationship with both schizophrenia and schizotypal personality disorder. Although it can occur in younger age groups, the condition may be more prevalent in older individuals.

## Culture-Related Diagnostic Issues

An individual's cultural and religious background must be taken into account in evaluating the possible presence of delusional disorder. The content of delusions also varies across cultural contexts.

## Functional Consequences of Delusional Disorder

The functional impairment is usually more circumscribed than that seen with other psychotic disorders, although in some cases, the impairment may be substantial and include poor occupational functioning and social isolation. When poor psychosocial functioning is present, delusional beliefs themselves often play a significant role. A common characteristic of individuals with delusional disorder is the apparent normality of their behavior and appearance when their delusional ideas are not being discussed or acted on.

## Differential Diagnosis

**Obsessive-compulsive and related disorders.**    If an individual with obsessive-compulsive disorder is completely convinced that his or her obsessive-compulsive disorder beliefs are true, then the diagnosis of obsessive-compulsive disorder, with absent insight/delusional beliefs specifier, should be given rather than a diagnosis of delusional disorder. Similarly, if an individual with body dysmorphic disorder is completely convinced that his or her body dysmorphic disorder beliefs are true, then the diagnosis of body dysmorphic disorder, with absent insight/delusional beliefs specifier, should be given rather than a diagnosis of delusional disorder.

**Delirium, major neurocognitive disorder, psychotic disorder due to another medical condition, and substance/medication-induced psychotic disorder.**    Individuals with these disorders may present with symptoms that suggest delusional disorder. For example, simple persecutory delusions in the context of major neurocognitive disorder would be diagnosed as major neurocognitive disorder, with behavioral disturbance. A substance/medication-induced psychotic disorder cross-sectionally may be identical in symptomatology to delusional disorder but can be distinguished by the chronological relationship of substance use to the onset and remission of the delusional beliefs.

**Schizophrenia and schizophreniform disorder.**    Delusional disorder can be distinguished from schizophrenia and schizophreniform disorder by the absence of the other characteristic symptoms of the active phase of schizophrenia.

**Depressive and bipolar disorders and schizoaffective disorder.** These disorders may be distinguished from delusional disorder by the temporal relationship between the mood disturbance and the delusions and by the severity of the mood symptoms. If delusions occur exclusively during mood episodes, the diagnosis is depressive or bipolar disorder with psychotic features. Mood symptoms that meet full criteria for a mood episode can be superimposed on delusional disorder. Delusional disorder can be diagnosed only if the total duration of all mood episodes remains brief relative to the total duration of the delusional disturbance. If not, then a diagnosis of other specified or unspecified schizophrenia spectrum and other psychotic disorder accompanied by other specified depressive disorder, unspecified depressive disorder, other specified bipolar and related disorder, or unspecified bipolar and related disorder is appropriate.

# Brief Psychotic Disorder

## Diagnostic Criteria                                                    298.8 (F23)

A. Presence of one (or more) of the following symptoms. At least one of these must be (1), (2), or (3):

1. Delusions.
2. Hallucinations.
3. Disorganized speech (e.g., frequent derailment or incoherence).
4. Grossly disorganized or catatonic behavior.

**Note:** Do not include a symptom if it is a culturally sanctioned response.

B. Duration of an episode of the disturbance is at least 1 day but less than 1 month, with eventual full return to premorbid level of functioning.

C. The disturbance is not better explained by major depressive or bipolar disorder with psychotic features or another psychotic disorder such as schizophrenia or catatonia, and is not attributable to the physiological effects of a substance (e.g., a drug of abuse, a medication) or another medical condition.

*Specify* if:

**With marked stressor(s)** (brief reactive psychosis): If symptoms occur in response to events that, singly or together, would be markedly stressful to almost anyone in similar circumstances in the individual's culture.

**Without marked stressor(s):** If symptoms do not occur in response to events that, singly or together, would be markedly stressful to almost anyone in similar circumstances in the individual's culture.

**With peripartum onset:** If onset is during pregnancy or within 4 weeks postpartum.

*Specify* if:

**With catatonia** (refer to the criteria for catatonia associated with another mental disorder, [DSM-5] pp. 119–120, for definition)

**Coding note:** Use additional code 293.89 (F06.1) catatonia associated with brief psychotic disorder to indicate the presence of the comorbid catatonia.

*Specify* current severity:

Severity is rated by a quantitative assessment of the primary symptoms of psychosis, including delusions, hallucinations, disorganized speech, abnormal psychomotor behavior, and negative symptoms. Each of these symptoms may be rated for its current severity (most severe in the last 7 days) on a 5-point scale ranging from 0 (not present) to 4 (present and severe). (See Clinician-Rated Dimensions of Psychosis Symptom Severity in the chapter "Assessment Measures" [in DSM-5].)

**Note:** Diagnosis of brief psychotic disorder can be made without using this severity specifier.

## Diagnostic Features

The essential feature of brief psychotic disorder is a disturbance that involves the sudden onset of at least one of the following positive psychotic symptoms: delusions, hallucinations, disorganized speech (e.g., frequent derailment or incoherence), or grossly abnormal psychomotor behavior, including catatonia (Criterion A). *Sudden onset* is defined as change from a nonpsychotic state to a clearly psychotic state within 2 weeks, usually without a prodrome. An episode of the disturbance lasts at least 1 day but less than 1 month, and the individual eventually has a full return to the premorbid level of functioning (Criterion B). The disturbance is not better explained by a depressive or bipolar disorder with psychotic features, by schizoaffective disorder, or by schizophrenia and is not attributable to the physiological effects of a substance (e.g., a hallucinogen) or another medical condition (e.g., subdural hematoma) (Criterion C).

In addition to the five symptom domain areas identified in the diagnostic criteria, the assessment of cognition, depression, and mania symptom domains is vital for making critically important distinctions between the various schizophrenia spectrum and other psychotic disorders.

## Associated Features Supporting Diagnosis

Individuals with brief psychotic disorder typically experience emotional turmoil or overwhelming confusion. They may have rapid shifts from one intense affect to another. Although the disturbance is brief, the level of impairment may be severe, and supervision may be required to ensure that nutritional and hygienic needs are met and that the individual is protected from the consequences of poor judgment, cognitive impairment, or acting on the basis of delusions. There appears to be an increased risk of suicidal behavior, particularly during the acute episode.

## Prevalence

In the United States, brief psychotic disorder may account for 9% of cases of first-onset psychosis. Psychotic disturbances that meet Criteria A and C, but not Criterion B, for brief psychotic disorder (i.e., duration of active symptoms is 1–6 months as opposed to remission within 1 month) are more common in developing countries than in developed countries. Brief psychotic disorder is twofold more common in females than in males.

## Development and Course

Brief psychotic disorder may appear in adolescence or early adulthood, and onset can occur across the lifespan, with the average age at onset being the mid 30s. By definition, a diagnosis of brief psychotic disorder requires a full remission of all symptoms and an eventual full return to the premorbid level of functioning within 1 month of the onset of the disturbance. In some individuals, the duration of psychotic symptoms may be quite brief (e.g., a few days).

## Risk and Prognostic Factors

**Temperamental.** Preexisting personality disorders and traits (e.g., schizotypal personality disorder; borderline personality disorder; or traits in the psychoticism domain, such as perceptual dysregulation, and the negative affectivity domain, such as suspiciousness) may predispose the individual to the development of the disorder.

## Culture-Related Diagnostic Issues

It is important to distinguish symptoms of brief psychotic disorder from culturally sanctioned response patterns. For example, in some religious ceremonies, an individual may report hearing voices, but these do not generally persist and are not perceived as abnormal by most members of the individual's community. In addition, cultural and religious background must be taken into account when considering whether beliefs are delusional.

## Functional Consequences of Brief Psychotic Disorder

Despite high rates of relapse, for most individuals, outcome is excellent in terms of social functioning and symptomatology.

## Differential Diagnosis

**Other medical conditions.** A variety of medical disorders can manifest with psychotic symptoms of short duration. Psychotic disorder due to another medical condition or a delirium is diagnosed when there is evidence from the history, physical examination, or laboratory tests that the delusions or hallucinations are the direct physiological consequence of a specific medical condition (e.g., Cushing's syndrome, brain tumor) (see "Psychotic Disorder Due to Another Medical Condition" later in this chapter).

**Substance-related disorders.** Substance/medication-induced psychotic disorder, substance-induced delirium, and substance intoxication are distinguished from brief psychotic disorder by the fact that a substance (e.g., a drug of abuse, a medication, exposure to a toxin) is judged to be etiologically related to the psychotic symptoms (see "Substance/Medication-Induced Psychotic Disorder" later in this chapter). Laboratory tests, such as a urine drug screen or a blood alcohol level, may be helpful in making this determination, as may a careful history of substance use with attention to temporal relationships between substance intake and onset of the symptoms and to the nature of the substance being used.

**Depressive and bipolar disorders.**   The diagnosis of brief psychotic disorder cannot be made if the psychotic symptoms are better explained by a mood episode (i.e., the psychotic symptoms occur exclusively during a full major depressive, manic, or mixed episode).

**Other psychotic disorders.**   If the psychotic symptoms persist for 1 month or longer, the diagnosis is either schizophreniform disorder, delusional disorder, depressive disorder with psychotic features, bipolar disorder with psychotic features, or other specified or unspecified schizophrenia spectrum and other psychotic disorder, depending on the other symptoms in the presentation. The differential diagnosis between brief psychotic disorder and schizophreniform disorder is difficult when the psychotic symptoms have remitted before 1 month in response to successful treatment with medication. Careful attention should be given to the possibility that a recurrent disorder (e.g., bipolar disorder, recurrent acute exacerbations of schizophrenia) may be responsible for any recurring psychotic episodes.

**Malingering and factitious disorders.**   An episode of factitious disorder, with predominantly psychological signs and symptoms, may have the appearance of brief psychotic disorder, but in such cases there is evidence that the symptoms are intentionally produced. When malingering involves apparently psychotic symptoms, there is usually evidence that the illness is being feigned for an understandable goal.

**Personality disorders.**   In certain individuals with personality disorders, psychosocial stressors may precipitate brief periods of psychotic symptoms. These symptoms are usually transient and do not warrant a separate diagnosis. If psychotic symptoms persist for at least 1 day, an additional diagnosis of brief psychotic disorder may be appropriate.

# Schizophreniform Disorder

Diagnostic Criteria                                          **295.40 (F20.81)**

A. Two (or more) of the following, each present for a significant portion of time during a 1-month period (or less if successfully treated). At least one of these must be (1), (2), or (3):
   1. Delusions.
   2. Hallucinations.
   3. Disorganized speech (e.g., frequent derailment or incoherence).
   4. Grossly disorganized or catatonic behavior.
   5. Negative symptoms (i.e., diminished emotional expression or avolition).
B. An episode of the disorder lasts at least 1 month but less than 6 months. When the diagnosis must be made without waiting for recovery, it should be qualified as "provisional."
C. Schizoaffective disorder and depressive or bipolar disorder with psychotic features have been ruled out because either 1) no major depressive or manic episodes have occurred concurrently with the active-phase symptoms, or 2) if mood episodes have occurred during active-phase symptoms, they have been present for a minority of the total duration of the active and residual periods of the illness.

D.  The disturbance is not attributable to the physiological effects of a substance (e.g., a drug of abuse, a medication) or another medical condition.

*Specify* if:

**With good prognostic features:** This specifier requires the presence of at least two of the following features: onset of prominent psychotic symptoms within 4 weeks of the first noticeable change in usual behavior or functioning; confusion or perplexity; good premorbid social and occupational functioning; and absence of blunted or flat affect.

**Without good prognostic features:** This specifier is applied if two or more of the above features have not been present.

*Specify* if:

**With catatonia** (refer to the criteria for catatonia associated with another mental disorder, [DSM-5] pp. 119–120, for definition).

   **Coding note:** Use additional code 293.89 (F06.1) catatonia associated with schizophreniform disorder to indicate the presence of the comorbid catatonia.

*Specify* current severity:

Severity is rated by a quantitative assessment of the primary symptoms of psychosis, including delusions, hallucinations, disorganized speech, abnormal psychomotor behavior, and negative symptoms. Each of these symptoms may be rated for its current severity (most severe in the last 7 days) on a 5-point scale ranging from 0 (not present) to 4 (present and severe). (See Clinician-Rated Dimensions of Psychosis Symptom Severity in the chapter "Assessment Measures" [in DSM-5].)

**Note:** Diagnosis of schizophreniform disorder can be made without using this severity specifier.

---

**Note:** For additional information on Associated Features Supporting Diagnosis, Development and Course (age-related factors), Culture-Related Diagnostic Issues, Gender-Related Diagnostic Issues, Differential Diagnosis, and Comorbidity, see the corresponding sections in schizophrenia.

## Diagnostic Features

The characteristic symptoms of schizophreniform disorder are identical to those of schizophrenia (Criterion A). Schizophreniform disorder is distinguished by its difference in duration: the total duration of the illness, including prodromal, active, and residual phases, is at least 1 month but less than 6 months (Criterion B). The duration requirement for schizophreniform disorder is intermediate between that for brief psychotic disorder, which lasts more than 1 day and remits by 1 month, and schizophrenia, which lasts for at least 6 months. The diagnosis of schizophreniform disorder is made under two conditions: 1) when an episode of illness lasts between 1 and 6 months and the individual has already recovered, and 2) when an individual is symptomatic for less than the 6 months' duration required for the diagnosis of schizophrenia but has not yet recovered. In this case, the diagnosis should be noted as "schizophreniform disorder (provisional)" because it is uncertain if the individual will recover from the disturbance within the 6-month period. If the disturbance persists beyond 6 months, the diagnosis should be changed to schizophrenia.

Another distinguishing feature of schizophreniform disorder is the lack of a criterion requiring impaired social and occupational functioning. While such impairments may potentially be present, they are not necessary for a diagnosis of schizophreniform disorder.

In addition to the five symptom domain areas identified in the diagnostic criteria, the assessment of cognition, depression, and mania symptom domains is vital for making critically important distinctions between the various schizophrenia spectrum and other psychotic disorders.

## Associated Features Supporting Diagnosis

As with schizophrenia, currently there are no laboratory or psychometric tests for schizophreniform disorder. There are multiple brain regions where neuroimaging, neuropathological, and neurophysiological research has indicated abnormalities, but none are diagnostic.

## Prevalence

Incidence of schizophreniform disorder across sociocultural settings is likely similar to that observed in schizophrenia. In the United States and other developed countries, the incidence is low, possibly fivefold less than that of schizophrenia. In developing countries, the incidence may be higher, especially for the specifier "with good prognostic features"; in some of these settings schizophreniform disorder may be as common as schizophrenia.

## Development and Course

The development of schizophreniform disorder is similar to that of schizophrenia. About one-third of individuals with an initial diagnosis of schizophreniform disorder (provisional) recover within the 6-month period and schizophreniform disorder is their final diagnosis. The majority of the remaining two-thirds of individuals will eventually receive a diagnosis of schizophrenia or schizoaffective disorder.

## Risk and Prognostic Factors

**Genetic and physiological.**   Relatives of individuals with schizophreniform disorder have an increased risk for schizophrenia.

## Functional Consequences of Schizophreniform Disorder

For the majority of individuals with schizophreniform disorder who eventually receive a diagnosis of schizophrenia or schizoaffective disorder, the functional consequences are similar to the consequences of those disorders. Most individuals experience dysfunction in several areas of daily functioning, such as school or work, interpersonal relationships, and self-care. Individuals who recover from schizophreniform disorder have better functional outcomes.

## Differential Diagnosis

**Other mental disorders and medical conditions.** A wide variety of mental and medical conditions can manifest with psychotic symptoms that must be considered in the differential diagnosis of schizophreniform disorder. These include psychotic disorder due to another medical condition or its treatment; delirium or major neurocognitive disorder; substance/medication-induced psychotic disorder or delirium; depressive or bipolar disorder with psychotic features; schizoaffective disorder; other specified or unspecified bipolar and related disorder; depressive or bipolar disorder with catatonic features; schizophrenia; brief psychotic disorder; delusional disorder; other specified or unspecified schizophrenia spectrum and other psychotic disorder; schizotypal, schizoid, or paranoid personality disorders; autism spectrum disorder; disorders presenting in childhood with disorganized speech; attention-deficit/hyperactivity disorder; obsessive-compulsive disorder; posttraumatic stress disorder; and traumatic brain injury.

Since the diagnostic criteria for schizophreniform disorder and schizophrenia differ primarily in duration of illness, the discussion of the differential diagnosis of schizophrenia also applies to schizophreniform disorder.

**Brief psychotic disorder.** Schizophreniform disorder differs in duration from brief psychotic disorder, which has a duration of less than 1 month.

# Schizophrenia

Diagnostic Criteria | **295.90 (F20.9)**

A. Two (or more) of the following, each present for a significant portion of time during a 1-month period (or less if successfully treated). At least one of these must be (1), (2), or (3):

1. Delusions.
2. Hallucinations.
3. Disorganized speech (e.g., frequent derailment or incoherence).
4. Grossly disorganized or catatonic behavior.
5. Negative symptoms (i.e., diminished emotional expression or avolition).

B. For a significant portion of the time since the onset of the disturbance, level of functioning in one or more major areas, such as work, interpersonal relations, or self-care, is markedly below the level achieved prior to the onset (or when the onset is in childhood or adolescence, there is failure to achieve expected level of interpersonal, academic, or occupational functioning).

C. Continuous signs of the disturbance persist for at least 6 months. This 6-month period must include at least 1 month of symptoms (or less if successfully treated) that meet Criterion A (i.e., active-phase symptoms) and may include periods of prodromal or residual symptoms. During these prodromal or residual periods, the signs of the disturbance may be manifested by only negative symptoms or by two or more symptoms listed in Criterion A present in an attenuated form (e.g., odd beliefs, unusual perceptual experiences).

D.  Schizoaffective disorder and depressive or bipolar disorder with psychotic features have been ruled out because either 1) no major depressive or manic episodes have occurred concurrently with the active-phase symptoms, or 2) if mood episodes have occurred during active-phase symptoms, they have been present for a minority of the total duration of the active and residual periods of the illness.

E.  The disturbance is not attributable to the physiological effects of a substance (e.g., a drug of abuse, a medication) or another medical condition.

F.  If there is a history of autism spectrum disorder or a communication disorder of childhood onset, the additional diagnosis of schizophrenia is made only if prominent delusions or hallucinations, in addition to the other required symptoms of schizophrenia, are also present for at least 1 month (or less if successfully treated).

*Specify* if:

The following course specifiers are only to be used after a 1-year duration of the disorder and if they are not in contradiction to the diagnostic course criteria.

**First episode, currently in acute episode:** First manifestation of the disorder meeting the defining diagnostic symptom and time criteria. An *acute episode* is a time period in which the symptom criteria are fulfilled.

**First episode, currently in partial remission:** *Partial remission* is a period of time during which an improvement after a previous episode is maintained and in which the defining criteria of the disorder are only partially fulfilled.

**First episode, currently in full remission:** *Full remission* is a period of time after a previous episode during which no disorder-specific symptoms are present.

**Multiple episodes, currently in acute episode:** Multiple episodes may be determined after a minimum of two episodes (i.e., after a first episode, a remission and a minimum of one relapse).

**Multiple episodes, currently in partial remission**

**Multiple episodes, currently in full remission**

**Continuous:** Symptoms fulfilling the diagnostic symptom criteria of the disorder are remaining for the majority of the illness course, with subthreshold symptom periods being very brief relative to the overall course.

**Unspecified**

*Specify* if:

**With catatonia** (refer to the criteria for catatonia associated with another mental disorder, [DSM-5] pp. 119–120, for definition).

**Coding note:** Use additional code 293.89 (F06.1) catatonia associated with schizophrenia to indicate the presence of the comorbid catatonia.

*Specify* current severity:

Severity is rated by a quantitative assessment of the primary symptoms of psychosis, including delusions, hallucinations, disorganized speech, abnormal psychomotor behavior, and negative symptoms. Each of these symptoms may be rated for its current severity (most severe in the last 7 days) on a 5-point scale ranging from 0 (not present) to 4 (present and severe). (See Clinician-Rated Dimensions of Psychosis Symptom Severity in the chapter "Assessment Measures" [in DSM-5].)

**Note:** Diagnosis of schizophrenia can be made without using this severity specifier.

# Diagnostic Features

The characteristic symptoms of schizophrenia involve a range of cognitive, behavioral, and emotional dysfunctions, but no single symptom is pathognomonic of the disorder. The diagnosis involves the recognition of a constellation of signs and symptoms associated with impaired occupational or social functioning. Individuals with the disorder will vary substantially on most features, as schizophrenia is a heterogeneous clinical syndrome.

At least two Criterion A symptoms must be present for a significant portion of time during a 1-month period or longer. At least one of these symptoms must be the clear presence of delusions (Criterion A1), hallucinations (Criterion A2), or disorganized speech (Criterion A3). Grossly disorganized or catatonic behavior (Criterion A4) and negative symptoms (Criterion A5) may also be present. In those situations in which the active-phase symptoms remit within a month in response to treatment, Criterion A is still met if the clinician estimates that they would have persisted in the absence of treatment.

Schizophrenia involves impairment in one or more major areas of functioning (Criterion B). If the disturbance begins in childhood or adolescence, the expected level of function is not attained. Comparing the individual with unaffected siblings may be helpful. The dysfunction persists for a substantial period during the course of the disorder and does not appear to be a direct result of any single feature. Avolition (i.e., reduced drive to pursue goal-directed behavior; Criterion A5) is linked to the social dysfunction described under Criterion B. There is also strong evidence for a relationship between cognitive impairment (see the section "Associated Features Supporting Diagnosis" for this disorder) and functional impairment in individuals with schizophrenia.

Some signs of the disturbance must persist for a continuous period of at least 6 months (Criterion C). Prodromal symptoms often precede the active phase, and residual symptoms may follow it, characterized by mild or subthreshold forms of hallucinations or delusions. Individuals may express a variety of unusual or odd beliefs that are not of delusional proportions (e.g., ideas of reference or magical thinking); they may have unusual perceptual experiences (e.g., sensing the presence of an unseen person); their speech may be generally understandable but vague; and their behavior may be unusual but not grossly disorganized (e.g., mumbling in public). Negative symptoms are common in the prodromal and residual phases and can be severe. Individuals who had been socially active may become withdrawn from previous routines. Such behaviors are often the first sign of a disorder.

Mood symptoms and full mood episodes are common in schizophrenia and may be concurrent with active-phase symptomatology. However, as distinct from a psychotic mood disorder, a schizophrenia diagnosis requires the presence of delusions or hallucinations in the absence of mood episodes. In addition, mood episodes, taken in total, should be present for only a minority of the total duration of the active and residual periods of the illness.

In addition to the five symptom domain areas identified in the diagnostic criteria, the assessment of cognition, depression, and mania symptom domains is vital for making critically important distinctions between the various schizophrenia spectrum and other psychotic disorders.

## Associated Features Supporting Diagnosis

Individuals with schizophrenia may display inappropriate affect (e.g., laughing in the absence of an appropriate stimulus); a dysphoric mood that can take the form of depression, anxiety, or anger; a disturbed sleep pattern (e.g., daytime sleeping and nighttime activity); and a lack of interest in eating or food refusal. Depersonalization, derealization, and somatic concerns may occur and sometimes reach delusional proportions. Anxiety and phobias are common. Cognitive deficits in schizophrenia are common and are strongly linked to vocational and functional impairments. These deficits can include decrements in declarative memory, working memory, language function, and other executive functions, as well as slower processing speed. Abnormalities in sensory processing and inhibitory capacity, as well as reductions in attention, are also found. Some individuals with schizophrenia show social cognition deficits, including deficits in the ability to infer the intentions of other people (theory of mind), and may attend to and then interpret irrelevant events or stimuli as meaningful, perhaps leading to the generation of explanatory delusions. These impairments frequently persist during symptomatic remission.

Some individuals with psychosis may lack insight or awareness of their disorder (i.e., anosognosia). This lack of "insight" includes unawareness of symptoms of schizophrenia and may be present throughout the entire course of the illness. Unawareness of illness is typically a symptom of schizophrenia itself rather than a coping strategy. It is comparable to the lack of awareness of neurological deficits following brain damage, termed *anosognosia*. This symptom is the most common predictor of nonadherence to treatment, and it predicts higher relapse rates, increased number of involuntary treatments, poorer psychosocial functioning, aggression, and a poorer course of illness.

Hostility and aggression can be associated with schizophrenia, although spontaneous or random assault is uncommon. Aggression is more frequent for younger males and for individuals with a past history of violence, non-adherence with treatment, substance abuse, and impulsivity. It should be noted that the vast majority of persons with schizophrenia are not aggressive and are more frequently victimized than are individuals in the general population.

Currently, there are no radiological, laboratory, or psychometric tests for the disorder. Differences are evident in multiple brain regions between groups of healthy individuals and persons with schizophrenia, including evidence from neuroimaging, neuropathological, and neurophysiological studies. Differences are also evident in cellular architecture, white matter connectivity, and gray matter volume in a variety of regions such as the prefrontal and temporal cortices. Reduced overall brain volume has been observed, as well as increased brain volume reduction with age. Brain volume reductions with age are more pronounced in individuals with schizophrenia than in healthy individuals. Finally, individuals with schizophrenia appear to differ from individuals without the disorder in eye-tracking and electrophysiological indices.

Neurological soft signs common in individuals with schizophrenia include impairments in motor coordination, sensory integration, and motor sequencing of complex movements; left-right confusion; and disinhibition of associated movements. In addition, minor physical anomalies of the face and limbs may occur.

# Prevalence

The lifetime prevalence of schizophrenia appears to be approximately 0.3%–0.7%, although there is reported variation by race/ethnicity, across countries, and by geographic origin for immigrants and children of immigrants. The sex ratio differs across samples and populations: for example, an emphasis on negative symptoms and longer duration of disorder (associated with poorer outcome) shows higher incidence rates for males, whereas definitions allowing for the inclusion of more mood symptoms and brief presentations (associated with better outcome) show equivalent risks for both sexes.

# Development and Course

The psychotic features of schizophrenia typically emerge between the late teens and the mid-30s; onset prior to adolescence is rare. The peak age at onset for the first psychotic episode is in the early to mid-20s for males and in the late-20s for females. The onset may be abrupt or insidious, but the majority of individuals manifest a slow and gradual development of a variety of clinically significant signs and symptoms. Half of these individuals complain of depressive symptoms. Earlier age at onset has traditionally been seen as a predictor of worse prognosis. However, the effect of age at onset is likely related to gender, with males having worse premorbid adjustment, lower educational achievement, more prominent negative symptoms and cognitive impairment, and in general a worse outcome. Impaired cognition is common, and alterations in cognition are present during development and precede the emergence of psychosis, taking the form of stable cognitive impairments during adulthood. Cognitive impairments may persist when other symptoms are in remission and contribute to the disability of the disease.

The predictors of course and outcome are largely unexplained, and course and outcome may not be reliably predicted. The course appears to be favorable in about 20% of those with schizophrenia, and a small number of individuals are reported to recover completely. However, most individuals with schizophrenia still require formal or informal daily living supports, and many remain chronically ill, with exacerbations and remissions of active symptoms, while others have a course of progressive deterioration.

Psychotic symptoms tend to diminish over the life course, perhaps in association with normal age-related declines in dopamine activity. Negative symptoms are more closely related to prognosis than are positive symptoms and tend to be the most persistent. Furthermore, cognitive deficits associated with the illness may not improve over the course of the illness.

The essential features of schizophrenia are the same in childhood, but it is more difficult to make the diagnosis. In children, delusions and hallucinations may be less elaborate than in adults, and visual hallucinations are more common and should be distinguished from normal fantasy play. Disorganized speech occurs in many disorders with childhood onset (e.g., autism spectrum disorder), as does disorganized behavior (e.g., attention-deficit/hyperactivity disorder). These symptoms should not be attributed to schizophrenia without due consideration of the more common disorders of childhood. Childhood-onset cases tend to resemble poor-outcome adult cases, with gradual onset and prominent negative symptoms. Children who later receive the diagnosis of schizophrenia are more likely to have experienced nonspecific emotional-behavioral disturbances and psychopathology, intellectual and language alterations, and subtle motor delays.

Late-onset cases (i.e., onset after age 40 years) are overrepresented by females, who may have married. Often, the course is characterized by a predominance of psychotic symptoms with preservation of affect and social functioning. Such late-onset cases can still meet the diagnostic criteria for schizophrenia, but it is not yet clear whether this is the same condition as schizophrenia diagnosed prior to mid-life (e.g., prior to age 55 years).

## Risk and Prognostic Factors

**Environmental.** Season of birth has been linked to the incidence of schizophrenia, including late winter/early spring in some locations and summer for the deficit form of the disease. The incidence of schizophrenia and related disorders is higher for children growing up in an urban environment and for some minority ethnic groups.

**Genetic and physiological.** There is a strong contribution for genetic factors in determining risk for schizophrenia, although most individuals who have been diagnosed with schizophrenia have no family history of psychosis. Liability is conferred by a spectrum of risk alleles, common and rare, with each allele contributing only a small fraction to the total population variance. The risk alleles identified to date are also associated with other mental disorders, including bipolar disorder, depression, and autism spectrum disorder.

Pregnancy and birth complications with hypoxia and greater paternal age are associated with a higher risk of schizophrenia for the developing fetus. In addition, other prenatal and perinatal adversities, including stress, infection, malnutrition, maternal diabetes, and other medical conditions, have been linked with schizophrenia. However, the vast majority of offspring with these risk factors do not develop schizophrenia.

## Culture-Related Diagnostic Issues

Cultural and socioeconomic factors must be considered, particularly when the individual and the clinician do not share the same cultural and socioeconomic background. Ideas that appear to be delusional in one culture (e.g., witchcraft) may be commonly held in another. In some cultures, visual or auditory hallucinations with a religious content (e.g., hearing God's voice) are a normal part of religious experience. In addition, the assessment of disorganized speech may be made difficult by linguistic variation in narrative styles across cultures. The assessment of affect requires sensitivity to differences in styles of emotional expression, eye contact, and body language, which vary across cultures. If the assessment is conducted in a language that is different from the individual's primary language, care must be taken to ensure that alogia is not related to linguistic barriers. In certain cultures, distress may take the form of hallucinations or pseudo-hallucinations and overvalued ideas that may present clinically similar to true psychosis but are normative to the patient's subgroup.

## Gender-Related Diagnostic Issues

A number of features distinguish the clinical expression of schizophrenia in females and males. The general incidence of schizophrenia tends to be slightly lower in females, particularly among treated cases. The age at onset is later in females, with a second mid-life peak as described earlier (see the section "Development and Course" for this disorder). Symptoms tend to be more affect-laden among females, and there are more psychotic symptoms, as well as a greater propensity for psychotic symptoms to worsen in later life. Other symptom differences include less frequent negative symptoms and disorganization. Finally, social functioning tends to remain better preserved in females. There are, however, frequent exceptions to these general caveats.

## Suicide Risk

Approximately 5%–6% of individuals with schizophrenia die by suicide, about 20% attempt suicide on one or more occasions, and many more have significant suicidal ideation. Suicidal behavior is sometimes in response to command hallucinations to harm oneself or others. Suicide risk remains high over the whole lifespan for males and females, although it may be especially high for younger males with comorbid substance use. Other risk factors include having depressive symptoms or feelings of hopelessness and being unemployed, and the risk is higher, also, in the period after a psychotic episode or hospital discharge.

## Functional Consequences of Schizophrenia

Schizophrenia is associated with significant social and occupational dysfunction. Making educational progress and maintaining employment are frequently impaired by avolition or other disorder manifestations, even when the cognitive skills are sufficient for the tasks at hand. Most individuals are employed at a lower level than their parents, and most, particularly men, do not marry or have limited social contacts outside of their family.

## Differential Diagnosis

**Major depressive or bipolar disorder with psychotic or catatonic features.**   The distinction between schizophrenia and major depressive or bipolar disorder with psychotic features or with catatonia depends on the temporal relationship between the mood disturbance and the psychosis, and on the severity of the depressive or manic symptoms. If delusions or hallucinations occur exclusively during a major depressive or manic episode, the diagnosis is depressive or bipolar disorder with psychotic features.

**Schizoaffective disorder.**   A diagnosis of schizoaffective disorder requires that a major depressive or manic episode occur concurrently with the active-phase symptoms and that the mood symptoms be present for a majority of the total duration of the active periods.

**Schizophreniform disorder and brief psychotic disorder.**   These disorders are of shorter duration than schizophrenia as specified in Criterion C, which requires 6 months of symptoms. In schizophreniform disorder, the disturbance is present less than 6 months, and in brief psychotic disorder, symptoms are present at least 1 day but less than 1 month.

**Delusional disorder.**   Delusional disorder can be distinguished from schizophrenia by the absence of the other symptoms characteristic of schizophrenia (e.g., delusions, prominent auditory or visual hallucinations, disorganized speech, grossly disorganized or catatonic behavior, negative symptoms).

**Schizotypal personality disorder.**   Schizotypal personality disorder may be distinguished from schizophrenia by subthreshold symptoms that are associated with persistent personality features.

**Obsessive-compulsive disorder and body dysmorphic disorder.**   Individuals with obsessive-compulsive disorder and body dysmorphic disorder may present with poor or absent insight, and the preoccupations may reach delusional proportions. But these disorders are distinguished from schizophrenia by their prominent obsessions, compulsions, preoccupations with appearance or body odor, hoarding, or body-focused repetitive behaviors.

**Posttraumatic stress disorder.**   Posttraumatic stress disorder may include flashbacks that have a hallucinatory quality, and hypervigilance may reach paranoid proportions. But a traumatic event and characteristic symptom features relating to reliving or reacting to the event are required to make the diagnosis.

**Autism spectrum disorder or communication disorders.**   These disorders may also have symptoms resembling a psychotic episode but are distinguished by their respective deficits in social interaction with repetitive and restricted behaviors and other cognitive and communication deficits. An individual with autism spectrum disorder or communication disorder must have symptoms that meet full criteria for schizophrenia, with prominent hallucinations or delusions for at least 1 month, in order to be diagnosed with schizophrenia as a comorbid condition.

**Other mental disorders associated with a psychotic episode.**   The diagnosis of schizophrenia is made only when the psychotic episode is persistent and not attributable to the physiological effects of a substance or another medical condition. Individuals with a delirium or major or minor neurocognitive disorder may present with psychotic symptoms, but these would have a temporal relationship to the onset of cognitive changes consistent with those disorders. Individuals with substance/medication-induced psychotic disorder may present with symptoms characteristic of Criterion A for schizophrenia, but the substance/medication-induced psychotic disorder can usually be distinguished by the chronological relationship of substance use to the onset and remission of the psychosis in the absence of substance use.

## Comorbidity

Rates of comorbidity with substance-related disorders are high in schizophrenia. Over half of individuals with schizophrenia have tobacco use disorder and smoke cigarettes regularly. Comorbidity with anxiety disorders is increasingly recognized in schizophrenia. Rates of obsessive-compulsive disorder and panic disorder are elevated in individuals with schizophrenia compared with the general population. Schizotypal or paranoid personality disorder may sometimes precede the onset of schizophrenia.

Life expectancy is reduced in individuals with schizophrenia because of associated medical conditions. Weight gain, diabetes, metabolic syndrome, and cardiovascular and pulmonary disease are more common in schizophrenia than in the general population. Poor engagement in health maintenance behaviors (e.g., cancer screening, exercise) increases the risk of chronic disease, but other disorder factors, including medications, lifestyle, cigarette smoking, and diet, may also play a role. A shared vulnerability for psychosis and medical disorders may explain some of the medical comorbidity of schizophrenia.

# Schizoaffective Disorder

## Diagnostic Criteria

A. An uninterrupted period of illness during which there is a major mood episode (major depressive or manic) concurrent with Criterion A of schizophrenia.
   **Note:** The major depressive episode must include Criterion A1: Depressed mood.
B. Delusions or hallucinations for 2 or more weeks in the absence of a major mood episode (depressive or manic) during the lifetime duration of the illness.
C. Symptoms that meet criteria for a major mood episode are present for the majority of the total duration of the active and residual portions of the illness.
D. The disturbance is not attributable to the effects of a substance (e.g., a drug of abuse, a medication) or another medical condition.

*Specify* whether:
   **295.70 (F25.0) Bipolar type:** This subtype applies if a manic episode is part of the presentation. Major depressive episodes may also occur.
   **295.70 (F25.1) Depressive type:** This subtype applies if only major depressive episodes are part of the presentation.

*Specify* if:
   **With catatonia** (refer to the criteria for catatonia associated with another mental disorder, [DSM-5] pp. 119–120, for definition).
      **Coding note:** Use additional code 293.89 (F06.1) catatonia associated with schizoaffective disorder to indicate the presence of the comorbid catatonia.

*Specify* if:
The following course specifiers are only to be used after a 1-year duration of the disorder and if they are not in contradiction to the diagnostic course criteria.
   **First episode, currently in acute episode:** First manifestation of the disorder meeting the defining diagnostic symptom and time criteria. An *acute episode* is a time period in which the symptom criteria are fulfilled.
   **First episode, currently in partial remission:** *Partial remission* is a time period during which an improvement after a previous episode is maintained and in which the defining criteria of the disorder are only partially fulfilled.

**First episode, currently in full remission:** *Full remission* is a period of time after a previous episode during which no disorder-specific symptoms are present.

**Multiple episodes, currently in acute episode:** Multiple episodes may be determined after a minimum of two episodes (i.e., after a first episode, a remission and a minimum of one relapse).

**Multiple episodes, currently in partial remission**

**Multiple episodes, currently in full remission**

**Continuous:** Symptoms fulfilling the diagnostic symptom criteria of the disorder are remaining for the majority of the illness course, with subthreshold symptom periods being very brief relative to the overall course.

**Unspecified**

*Specify* current severity:

Severity is rated by a quantitative assessment of the primary symptoms of psychosis, including delusions, hallucinations, disorganized speech, abnormal psychomotor behavior, and negative symptoms. Each of these symptoms may be rated for its current severity (most severe in the last 7 days) on a 5-point scale ranging from 0 (not present) to 4 (present and severe). (See Clinician-Rated Dimensions of Psychosis Symptom Severity in the chapter "Assessment Measures" [in DSM-5].)

**Note:** Diagnosis of schizoaffective disorder can be made without using this severity specifier.

**Note:** For additional information on Development and Course (age-related factors), Risk and Prognostic Factors (environmental risk factors), Culture-Related Diagnostic Issues, and Gender-Related Diagnostic Issues, see the corresponding sections in schizophrenia, bipolar I and II disorders, and major depressive disorder in their respective chapters.

# Diagnostic Features

The diagnosis of schizoaffective disorder is based on the assessment of an uninterrupted period of illness during which the individual continues to display active or residual symptoms of psychotic illness. The diagnosis is usually, but not necessarily, made during the period of psychotic illness. At some time during the period, Criterion A for schizophrenia has to be met. Criteria B (social dysfunction) and F (exclusion of autism spectrum disorder or other communication disorder of childhood onset) for schizophrenia do not have to be met. In addition to meeting Criterion A for schizophrenia, there is a major mood episode (major depressive or manic) (Criterion A for schizoaffective disorder). Because loss of interest or pleasure is common in schizophrenia, to meet Criterion A for schizoaffective disorder, the major depressive episode must include pervasive depressed mood (i.e., the presence of markedly diminished interest or pleasure is not sufficient). Episodes of depression or mania are present for the majority of the total duration of the illness (i.e., after Criterion A has been met) (Criterion C for schizoaffective disorder). To separate schizoaffective disorder from a depressive or bipolar disorder with psychotic features, delusions or hallucinations must be present for at least 2 weeks in the absence of a major mood episode (depressive or manic) at some point during the lifetime duration of the illness (Criterion B for schizoaffective disorder). The symptoms must not be attributable to the effects of a substance or another medical condition (Criterion D for schizoaffective disorder).

Criterion C for schizoaffective disorder specifies that mood symptoms meeting criteria for a major mood episode must be present for the majority of the total duration of the active and residual portion of the illness. Criterion C requires the assessment of mood symptoms for the entire course of a psychotic illness, which differs from the criterion in DSM-IV, which required only an assessment of the current period of illness. If the mood symptoms are present for only a relatively brief period, the diagnosis is schizophrenia, not schizoaffective disorder. When deciding whether an individual's presentation meets Criterion C, the clinician should review the total duration of psychotic illness (i.e., both active and residual symptoms) and determine when significant mood symptoms (untreated or in need of treatment with antidepressant and/or mood-stabilizing medication) accompanied the psychotic symptoms. This determination requires sufficient historical information and clinical judgment. For example, an individual with a 4-year history of active and residual symptoms of schizophrenia develops depressive and manic episodes that, taken together, do not occupy more than 1 year during the 4-year history of psychotic illness. This presentation would not meet Criterion C.

In addition to the five symptom domain areas identified in the diagnostic criteria, the assessment of cognition, depression, and mania symptom domains is vital for making critically important distinctions between the various schizophrenia spectrum and other psychotic disorders.

## Associated Features Supporting Diagnosis

Occupational functioning is frequently impaired, but this is not a defining criterion (in contrast to schizophrenia). Restricted social contact and difficulties with self-care are associated with schizoaffective disorder, but negative symptoms may be less severe and less persistent than those seen in schizophrenia. Anosognosia (i.e., poor insight) is also common in schizoaffective disorder, but the deficits in insight may be less severe and pervasive than those in schizophrenia. Individuals with schizoaffective disorder may be at increased risk for later developing episodes of major depressive disorder or bipolar disorder if mood symptoms continue following the remission of symptoms meeting Criterion A for schizophrenia. There may be associated alcohol and other substance-related disorders.

There are no tests or biological measures that can assist in making the diagnosis of schizoaffective disorder. Whether schizoaffective disorder differs from schizophrenia with regard to associated features such as structural or functional brain abnormalities, cognitive deficits, or genetic risk factors is not clear.

## Prevalence

Schizoaffective disorder appears to be about one-third as common as schizophrenia. Lifetime prevalence of schizoaffective disorder is estimated to be 0.3%. The incidence of schizoaffective disorder is higher in females than in males, mainly due to an increased incidence of the depressive type among females.

## Development and Course

The typical age at onset of schizoaffective disorder is early adulthood, although onset can occur anywhere from adolescence to late in life. A significant number of individuals diagnosed with another psychotic illness initially will receive the diagnosis schizoaffective disorder later when the pattern of mood episodes has become more apparent. With the current diagnostic Criterion C, it is expected that the diagnosis for some individuals will convert from schizoaffective disorder to another disorder as mood symptoms become less prominent. The prognosis for schizoaffective disorder is somewhat better than the prognosis for schizophrenia but worse than the prognosis for mood disorders.

Schizoaffective disorder may occur in a variety of temporal patterns. The following is a typical pattern: An individual may have pronounced auditory hallucinations and persecutory delusions for 2 months before the onset of a prominent major depressive episode. The psychotic symptoms and the full major depressive episode are then present for 3 months. Then, the individual recovers completely from the major depressive episode, but the psychotic symptoms persist for another month before they too disappear. During this period of illness, the individual's symptoms concurrently met criteria for a major depressive episode and Criterion A for schizophrenia, and during this same period of illness, auditory hallucinations and delusions were present both before and after the depressive phase. The total period of illness lasted for about 6 months, with psychotic symptoms alone present during the initial 2 months, both depressive and psychotic symptoms present during the next 3 months, and psychotic symptoms alone present during the last month. In this instance, the duration of the depressive episode was not brief relative to the total duration of the psychotic disturbance, and thus the presentation qualifies for a diagnosis of schizoaffective disorder.

The expression of psychotic symptoms across the lifespan is variable. Depressive or manic symptoms can occur before the onset of psychosis, during acute psychotic episodes, during residual periods, and after cessation of psychosis. For example, an individual might present with prominent mood symptoms during the prodromal stage of schizophrenia. This pattern is not necessarily indicative of schizoaffective disorder, since it is the co-occurrence of psychotic and mood symptoms that is diagnostic. For an individual with symptoms that clearly meet the criteria for schizoaffective disorder but who on further follow-up only presents with residual psychotic symptoms (such as subthreshold psychosis and/or prominent negative symptoms), the diagnosis may be changed to schizophrenia, as the total proportion of psychotic illness compared with mood symptoms becomes more prominent. Schizoaffective disorder, bipolar type, may be more common in young adults, whereas schizoaffective disorder, depressive type, may be more common in older adults.

## Risk and Prognostic Factors

**Genetic and physiological.**    Among individuals with schizophrenia, there may be an increased risk for schizoaffective disorder in first-degree relatives. The risk for schizoaffective disorder may be increased among individuals who have a first-degree relative with schizophrenia, bipolar disorder, or schizoaffective disorder.

## Culture-Related Diagnostic Issues

Cultural and socioeconomic factors must be considered, particularly when the individual and the clinician do not share the same cultural and economic background. Ideas that appear to be delusional in one culture (e.g., witchcraft) may be commonly held in another. There is also some evidence in the literature for the overdiagnosis of schizophrenia compared with schizoaffective disorder in African American and Hispanic populations, so care must be taken to ensure a culturally appropriate evaluation that includes both psychotic and affective symptoms.

## Suicide Risk

The lifetime risk of suicide for schizophrenia and schizoaffective disorder is 5%, and the presence of depressive symptoms is correlated with a higher risk for suicide. There is evidence that suicide rates are higher in North American populations than in European, Eastern European, South American, and Indian populations of individuals with schizophrenia or schizoaffective disorder.

## Functional Consequences of Schizoaffective Disorder

Schizoaffective disorder is associated with social and occupational dysfunction, but dysfunction is not a diagnostic criterion (as it is for schizophrenia), and there is substantial variability between individuals diagnosed with schizoaffective disorder.

## Differential Diagnosis

**Other mental disorders and medical conditions.**   A wide variety of psychiatric and medical conditions can manifest with psychotic and mood symptoms that must be considered in the differential diagnosis of schizoaffective disorder. These include psychotic disorder due to another medical condition; delirium; major neurocognitive disorder; substance/medication-induced psychotic disorder or neurocognitive disorder; bipolar disorders with psychotic features; major depressive disorder with psychotic features; depressive or bipolar disorders with catatonic features; schizotypal, schizoid, or paranoid personality disorder; brief psychotic disorder; schizophreniform disorder; schizophrenia; delusional disorder; and other specified and unspecified schizophrenia spectrum and other psychotic disorders. Medical conditions and substance use can present with a combination of psychotic and mood symptoms, and thus psychotic disorder due to another medical condition needs to be excluded. Distinguishing schizoaffective disorder from schizophrenia and from depressive and bipolar disorders with psychotic features is often difficult. Criterion C is designed to separate schizoaffective disorder from schizophrenia, and Criterion B is designed to distinguish schizoaffective disorder from a depressive or bipolar disorder with psychotic features. More specifically, schizoaffective disorder can be distinguished from a depressive or bipolar disorder with psychotic features due to the presence of prominent delusions and/or hallucinations for at least 2 weeks in the absence of a major mood episode. In contrast, in depressive or bipolar disorders with psychotic features, the psychotic features primarily occur during the mood episode(s). Because the relative proportion of mood to psychotic symptoms may change over time, the appropriate diagnosis may change from and to schizoaffective disorder (e.g., a diagnosis of schizoaffective disorder for a severe and prominent major depressive episode lasting 3 months during the first 6 months of a persistent psychotic illness would be changed to schizophrenia if active psychotic or prominent residual symptoms persist over several years without a recurrence of another mood episode).

**Psychotic disorder due to another medical condition.**   Other medical conditions and substance use can manifest with a combination of psychotic and mood symptoms, and thus psychotic disorder due to another medical condition needs to be excluded.

**Schizophrenia, bipolar, and depressive disorders.**   Distinguishing schizoaffective disorder from schizophrenia and from depressive and bipolar disorders with psychotic features is often difficult. Criterion C is designed to separate schizoaffective disorder from schizophrenia, and Criterion B is designed to distinguish schizoaffective disorder from a depressive or bipolar disorder with psychotic features. More specifically, schizoaffective disorder can be distinguished from a depressive or bipolar disorder with psychotic features based on the presence of prominent delusions and/ or hallucinations for at least 2 weeks in the absence of a major mood episode. In contrast, in depressive or bipolar disorder with psychotic features, the psychotic features primarily occur during the mood episode(s). Because the relative proportion of mood to psychotic symptoms may change over time, the appropriate diagnosis may change from and to schizoaffective disorder. (For example, a diagnosis of schizoaffective disorder for a severe and prominent major depressive episode lasting 3 months during the first 6 months of a chronic psychotic illness would be changed to schizophrenia if active psychotic or prominent residual symptoms persist over several years without a recurrence of another mood episode.)

## Comorbidity

Many individuals diagnosed with schizoaffective disorder are also diagnosed with other mental disorders, especially substance use disorders and anxiety disorders. Similarly, the incidence of medical conditions is increased above base rate for the general population and leads to decreased life expectancy.

# Substance/Medication-Induced Psychotic Disorder

## Diagnostic Criteria

A. Presence of one or both of the following symptoms:
   1. Delusions.
   2. Hallucinations.

B. There is evidence from the history, physical examination, or laboratory findings of both (1) and (2):
   1. The symptoms in Criterion A developed during or soon after substance intoxication or withdrawal or after exposure to a medication.
   2. The involved substance/medication is capable of producing the symptoms in Criterion A.

C. The disturbance is not better explained by a psychotic disorder that is not substance/medication-induced. Such evidence of an independent psychotic disorder could include the following:

> The symptoms preceded the onset of the substance/medication use; the symptoms persist for a substantial period of time (e.g., about 1 month) after the cessation of acute withdrawal or severe intoxication; or there is other evidence of an independent non-substance/medication-induced psychotic disorder (e.g., a history of recurrent non-substance/medication-related episodes).

D. The disturbance does not occur exclusively during the course of a delirium.

E. The disturbance causes clinically significant distress or impairment in social, occupational, or other important areas of functioning.

**Note:** This diagnosis should be made instead of a diagnosis of substance intoxication or substance withdrawal only when the symptoms in Criterion A predominate in the clinical picture and when they are sufficiently severe to warrant clinical attention.

**Coding note:** The ICD-9-CM and ICD-10-CM codes for the [specific substance/medication]-induced psychotic disorders are indicated in the table below. Note that the ICD-10-CM code depends on whether or not there is a comorbid substance use disorder present for the same class of substance. If a mild substance use disorder is comorbid with the substance-induced psychotic disorder, the 4th position character is "1," and the clinician should record "mild [substance] use disorder" before the substance-induced psychotic disorder (e.g., "mild cocaine use disorder with cocaine-induced psychotic disorder"). If a moderate or severe substance use disorder is comorbid with the substance-induced psychotic disorder, the 4th position character is "2," and the clinician should record "moderate [substance] use disorder" or "severe [substance] use disorder," depending on the severity of the comorbid substance use disorder. If there is no comorbid substance use disorder (e.g., after a one-time heavy use of the substance), then the 4th position character is "9," and the clinician should record only the substance-induced psychotic disorder.

| | | ICD-10-CM | | |
|---|---|---|---|---|
| | ICD-9-CM | With use disorder, mild | With use disorder, moderate or severe | Without use disorder |
| Alcohol | 291.9 | F10.159 | F10.259 | F10.959 |
| Cannabis | 292.9 | F12.159 | F12.259 | F12.959 |
| Phencyclidine | 292.9 | F16.159 | F16.259 | F16.959 |
| Other hallucinogen | 292.9 | F16.159 | F16.259 | F16.959 |
| Inhalant | 292.9 | F18.159 | F18.259 | F18.959 |
| Sedative, hypnotic, or anxiolytic | 292.9 | F13.159 | F13.259 | F13.959 |
| Amphetamine (or other stimulant) | 292.9 | F15.159 | F15.259 | F15.959 |
| Cocaine | 292.9 | F14.159 | F14.259 | F14.959 |
| Other (or unknown) substance | 292.9 | F19.159 | F19.259 | F19.959 |

*Specify* if (see Table 1 in the chapter "Substance-Related and Addictive Disorders" [in DSM-5] for diagnoses associated with substance class):

**With onset during intoxication:** If the criteria are met for intoxication with the substance and the symptoms develop during intoxication.

**With onset during withdrawal:** If the criteria are met for withdrawal from the substance and the symptoms develop during, or shortly after, withdrawal.

*Specify* current severity:

Severity is rated by a quantitative assessment of the primary symptoms of psychosis, including delusions, hallucinations, abnormal psychomotor behavior, and negative symptoms. Each of these symptoms may be rated for its current severity (most severe in the last 7 days) on a 5-point scale ranging from 0 (not present) to 4 (present and severe). (See Clinician-Rated Dimensions of Psychosis Symptom Severity in the chapter "Assessment Measures" [in DSM-5].)

**Note:** Diagnosis of substance/medication-induced psychotic disorder can be made without using this severity specifier.

# Recording Procedures

**ICD-9-CM.** The name of the substance/medication-induced psychotic disorder begins with the specific substance (e.g., cocaine, dexamethasone) that is presumed to be causing the delusions or hallucinations. The diagnostic code is selected from the table included in the criteria set, which is based on the drug class. For substances that do not fit into any of the classes (e.g., dexamethasone), the code for "other substance" should be used; and in cases in which a substance is judged to be an etiological factor but the specific class of substance is unknown, the category "unknown substance" should be used.

The name of the disorder is followed by the specification of onset (i.e., onset during intoxication, onset during withdrawal). Unlike the recording procedures for ICD-10-CM, which combine the substance-induced disorder and substance use disorder into a single code, for ICD-9-CM a separate diagnostic code is given for the substance use disorder. For example, in the case of delusions occurring during intoxication in a man with a severe cocaine use disorder, the diagnosis is 292.9 cocaine-induced psychotic disorder, with onset during intoxication. An additional diagnosis of 304.20 severe cocaine use disorder is also given. When more than one substance is judged to play a significant role in the development of psychotic symptoms, each should be listed separately (e.g., 292.9 cannabis-induced psychotic disorder with onset during intoxication, with severe cannabis use disorder; 292.9 phencyclidine-induced psychotic disorder, with onset during intoxication, with mild phencyclidine use disorder).

**ICD-10-CM.** The name of the substance/medication-induced psychotic disorder begins with the specific substance (e.g., cocaine, dexamethasone) that is presumed to be causing the delusions or hallucinations. The diagnostic code is selected from the table included in the criteria set, which is based on the drug class and presence or absence of a comorbid substance use disorder. For substances that do not fit into any of the classes (e.g., dexamethasone), the code for "other substance" with no comorbid substance use should be used; and in cases in which a substance is judged to be an etiological factor but the specific class of substance is unknown, the category "unknown substance" with no comorbid substance use should be used.

When recording the name of the disorder, the comorbid substance use disorder (if any) is listed first, followed by the word "with," followed by the name of the substance-induced psychotic disorder, followed by the specification of onset (i.e., onset during intoxication, onset during withdrawal). For example, in the case of delusions occurring during intoxication in a man with a severe cocaine use disorder, the diagnosis is F14.259 severe cocaine use disorder with cocaine-induced psychotic disorder, with onset during intoxication. A separate diagnosis of the comorbid severe cocaine use disorder is not given. If the substance-induced psychotic disorder occurs without a comorbid substance use disorder (e.g., after a one-time heavy use of the substance), no accompanying substance use disorder is noted (e.g., F16.959 phencyclidine-induced psychotic disorder, with onset during intoxication). When more than one substance is judged to play a significant role in the development of psychotic symptoms, each should be listed separately (e.g., F12.259 severe cannabis use disorder with cannabis-induced psychotic disorder, with onset during intoxication; F16.159 mild phencyclidine use disorder with phencyclidine-induced psychotic disorder, with onset during intoxication).

## Diagnostic Features

The essential features of substance/medication-induced psychotic disorder are prominent delusions and/or hallucinations (Criterion A) that are judged to be due to the physiological effects of a substance/medication (i.e., a drug of abuse, a medication, or a toxin exposure) (Criterion B). Hallucinations that the individual realizes are substance/medication-induced are not included here and instead would be diagnosed as substance intoxication or substance withdrawal with the accompanying specifier "with perceptual disturbances" (applies to alcohol withdrawal; cannabis intoxication; sedative, hypnotic, or anxiolytic withdrawal; and stimulant intoxication).

A substance/medication-induced psychotic disorder is distinguished from a primary psychotic disorder by considering the onset, course, and other factors. For drugs of abuse, there must be evidence from the history, physical examination, or laboratory findings of substance use, intoxication, or withdrawal. Substance/medication-induced psychotic disorders arise during or soon after exposure to a medication or after substance intoxication or withdrawal but can persist for weeks, whereas primary psychotic disorders may precede the onset of substance/medication use or may occur during times of sustained abstinence. Once initiated, the psychotic symptoms may continue as long as the substance/medication use continues. Another consideration is the presence of features that are atypical of a primary psychotic disorder (e.g., atypical age at onset or course). For example, the appearance of delusions de novo in a person older than 35 years without a known history of a primary psychotic disorder should suggest the possibility of a substance/medication-induced psychotic disorder. Even a prior history of a primary psychotic disorder does not rule out the possibility of a substance/medication-induced psychotic disorder. In contrast, factors that suggest that the psychotic symptoms are better accounted for by a primary psychotic disorder include persistence of psychotic symptoms for a substantial period of time (i.e., a month or more) after the end of substance intoxication or acute substance withdrawal or after cessation of medication use; or a history of prior recurrent primary psychotic disorders. Other causes of psychotic symptoms must be considered even in an individual with substance intoxication or withdrawal, because substance use problems are not uncommon among individuals with non-substance/medication-induced psychotic disorders.

In addition to the four symptom domain areas identified in the diagnostic criteria, the assessment of cognition, depression, and mania symptom domains is vital for making critically important distinctions between the various schizophrenia spectrum and other psychotic disorders.

## Associated Features Supporting Diagnosis

Psychotic disorders can occur in association with intoxication with the following classes of substances: alcohol; cannabis; hallucinogens, including phencyclidine and related substances; inhalants; sedatives, hypnotics, and anxiolytics; stimulants (including cocaine); and other (or unknown) substances. Psychotic disorders can occur in association with withdrawal from the following classes of substances: alcohol; sedatives, hypnotics, and anxiolytics; and other (or unknown) substances.

Some of the medications reported to evoke psychotic symptoms include anesthetics and analgesics, anticholinergic agents, anticonvulsants, antihistamines, antihypertensive and cardiovascular medications, antimicrobial medications, antiparkinsonian medications, chemotherapeutic agents (e.g., cyclosporine, procarbazine), corticosteroids, gastrointestinal medications, muscle relaxants, nonsteroidal anti-inflammatory medications, other over-the-counter medications (e.g., phenylephrine, pseudoephedrine), antidepressant medication, and disulfiram. Toxins reported to induce psychotic symptoms include anticholinesterase, organophosphate insecticides, sarin and other nerve gases, carbon monoxide, carbon dioxide, and volatile substances such as fuel or paint.

## Prevalence

Prevalence of substance/medication-induced psychotic disorder in the general population is unknown. Between 7% and 25% of individuals presenting with a first episode of psychosis in different settings are reported to have substance/medication-induced psychotic disorder.

## Development and Course

The initiation of the disorder may vary considerably with the substance. For example, smoking a high dose of cocaine may produce psychosis within minutes, whereas days or weeks of high-dose alcohol or sedative use may be required to produce psychosis. Alcohol-induced psychotic disorder, with hallucinations, usually occurs only after prolonged, heavy ingestion of alcohol in individuals who have moderate to severe alcohol use disorder, and the hallucinations are generally auditory in nature.

Psychotic disorders induced by amphetamine and cocaine share similar clinical features. Persecutory delusions may rapidly develop shortly after use of amphetamine or a similarly acting sympathomimetic. The hallucination of bugs or vermin crawling in or under the skin (formication) can lead to scratching and extensive skin excoriations. Cannabis-induced psychotic disorder may develop shortly after high-dose cannabis use and usually involves persecutory delusions, marked anxiety, emotional lability, and depersonalization. The disorder usually remits within a day but in some cases may persist for a few days.

Substance/medication-induced psychotic disorder may at times persist when the offending agent is removed, such that it may be difficult initially to distinguish it from an independent psychotic disorder. Agents such as amphetamines, phencyclidine, and cocaine have been reported to evoke temporary psychotic states that can sometimes persist for weeks or longer despite removal of the agent and treatment with neuroleptic medication. In later life, polypharmacy for medical conditions and exposure to medications for parkinsonism, cardiovascular disease, and other medical disorders may be associated with a greater likelihood of psychosis induced by prescription medications as opposed to substances of abuse.

## Diagnostic Markers

With substances for which relevant blood levels are available (e.g., blood alcohol level, other quantifiable blood levels such as digoxin), the presence of a level consistent with toxicity may increase diagnostic certainty.

## Functional Consequences of Substance/Medication-Induced Psychotic Disorder

Substance/medication-induced psychotic disorder is typically severely disabling and consequently is observed most frequently in emergency rooms, as individuals are often brought to the acute-care setting when it occurs. However, the disability is typically self-limited and resolves upon removal of the offending agent.

## Differential Diagnosis

**Substance intoxication or substance withdrawal.** Individuals intoxicated with stimulants, cannabis, the opioid meperidine, or phencyclidine, or those withdrawing from alcohol or sedatives, may experience altered perceptions that they recognize as drug effects. If reality testing for these experiences remains intact (i.e., the individual recognizes that the perception is substance induced and neither believes in nor acts on it), the diagnosis is not substance/medication-induced psychotic disorder. Instead, substance intoxication or substance withdrawal, with perceptual disturbances, is diagnosed (e.g., cocaine intoxication, with perceptual disturbances). "Flashback" hallucinations that can occur long after the use of hallucinogens has stopped are diagnosed as hallucinogen persisting perception disorder. If substance/medication-induced psychotic symptoms occur exclusively during the course of a delirium, as in severe forms of alcohol withdrawal, the psychotic symptoms are considered to be an associated feature of the delirium and are not diagnosed separately. Delusions in the context of a major or mild neurocognitive disorder would be diagnosed as major or mild neurocognitive disorder, with behavioral disturbance.

**Primary psychotic disorder.** A substance/medication-induced psychotic disorder is distinguished from a primary psychotic disorder, such as schizophrenia, schizoaffective disorder, delusional disorder, brief psychotic disorder, other specified schizophrenia spectrum and other psychotic disorder, or unspecified schizophrenia spectrum and other psychotic disorder, by the fact that a substance is judged to be etiologically related to the symptoms.

**Psychotic disorder due to another medical condition.**   A substance/medication-induced psychotic disorder due to a prescribed treatment for a mental or medical condition must have its onset while the individual is receiving the medication (or during withdrawal, if there is a withdrawal syndrome associated with the medication). Because individuals with medical conditions often take medications for those conditions, the clinician must consider the possibility that the psychotic symptoms are caused by the physiological consequences of the medical condition rather than the medication, in which case psychotic disorder due to another medical condition is diagnosed. The history often provides the primary basis for such a judgment. At times, a change in the treatment for the medical condition (e.g., medication substitution or discontinuation) may be needed to determine empirically for that individual whether the medication is the causative agent. If the clinician has ascertained that the disturbance is attributable to both a medical condition and substance/medication use, both diagnoses (i.e., psychotic disorder due to another medical condition and substance/medication-induced psychotic disorder) may be given.

# Psychotic Disorder Due to Another Medical Condition

## Diagnostic Criteria

A. Prominent hallucinations or delusions.
B. There is evidence from the history, physical examination, or laboratory findings that the disturbance is the direct pathophysiological consequence of another medical condition.
C. The disturbance is not better explained by another mental disorder.
D. The disturbance does not occur exclusively during the course of a delirium.
E. The disturbance causes clinically significant distress or impairment in social, occupational, or other important areas of functioning.

*Specify* whether:
Code based on predominant symptom:
   **293.81 (F06.2) With delusions:** If delusions are the predominant symptom.
   **293.82 (F06.0) With hallucinations:** If hallucinations are the predominant symptom.

**Coding note:** Include the name of the other medical condition in the name of the mental disorder (e.g., 293.81 [F06.2] psychotic disorder due to malignant lung neoplasm, with delusions). The other medical condition should be coded and listed separately immediately before the psychotic disorder due to the medical condition (e.g., 162.9 [C34.90] malignant lung neoplasm; 293.81 [F06.2] psychotic disorder due to malignant lung neoplasm, with delusions).

*Specify* current severity:

Severity is rated by a quantitative assessment of the primary symptoms of psychosis, including delusions, hallucinations, abnormal psychomotor behavior, and negative symptoms. Each of these symptoms may be rated for its current severity (most severe in the last 7 days) on a 5-point scale ranging from 0 (not present) to 4 (present and severe). (See Clinician-Rated Dimensions of Psychosis Symptom Severity in the chapter "Assessment Measures" [in DSM-5].)

**Note:** Diagnosis of psychotic disorder due to another medical condition can be made without using this severity specifier.

## Specifiers

In addition to the symptom domain areas identified in the diagnostic criteria, the assessment of cognition, depression, and mania symptom domains is vital for making critically important distinctions between the various schizophrenia spectrum and other psychotic disorders.

## Diagnostic Features

The essential features of psychotic disorder due to another medical condition are prominent delusions or hallucinations that are judged to be attributable to the physiological effects of another medical condition and are not better explained by another mental disorder (e.g., the symptoms are not a psychologically mediated response to a severe medical condition, in which case a diagnosis of brief psychotic disorder, with marked stressor, would be appropriate).

Hallucinations can occur in any sensory modality (i.e., visual, olfactory, gustatory, tactile, or auditory), but certain etiological factors are likely to evoke specific hallucinatory phenomena. Olfactory hallucinations are suggestive of temporal lobe epilepsy. Hallucinations may vary from simple and unformed to highly complex and organized, depending on etiological and environmental factors. Psychotic disorder due to another medical condition is generally not diagnosed if the individual maintains reality testing for the hallucinations and appreciates that they result from the medical condition. Delusions may have a variety of themes, including somatic, grandiose, religious, and, most commonly, persecutory. On the whole, however, associations between delusions and particular medical conditions appear to be less specific than is the case for hallucinations.

In determining whether the psychotic disturbance is attributable to another medical condition, the presence of a medical condition must be identified and considered to be the etiology of the psychosis through a physiological mechanism. Although there are no infallible guidelines for determining whether the relationship between the psychotic disturbance and the medical condition is etiological, several considerations provide some guidance. One consideration is the presence of a temporal association between the onset, exacerbation, or remission of the medical condition and that of the psychotic disturbance. A second consideration is the presence of features that are atypical for a psychotic disorder (e.g., atypical age at onset or presence of visual or olfactory hallucinations). The disturbance must also be distinguished from a substance/medication-induced psychotic disorder or another mental disorder (e.g., an adjustment disorder).

## Associated Features Supporting Diagnosis

The temporal association of the onset or exacerbation of the medical condition offers the greatest diagnostic certainty that the delusions or hallucinations are attributable to a medical condition. Additional factors may include concomitant treatments for the underlying medical condition that confer a risk for psychosis independently, such as steroid treatment for autoimmune disorders.

## Prevalence

Prevalence rates for psychotic disorder due to another medical condition are difficult to estimate given the wide variety of underlying medical etiologies. Lifetime prevalence has been estimated to range from 0.21% to 0.54%. When the prevalence findings are stratified by age group, individuals older than 65 years have a significantly greater prevalence of 0.74% compared with those in younger age groups. Rates of psychosis also vary according to the underlying medical condition; conditions most commonly associated with psychosis include untreated endocrine and metabolic disorders, autoimmune disorders (e.g., systemic lupus erythematosus, N-methyl-D-aspartate (NMDA) receptor autoimmune encephalitis), or temporal lobe epilepsy. Psychosis due to epilepsy has been further differentiated into ictal, postictal, and interictal psychosis. The most common of these is postictal psychosis, observed in 2%–7.8% of epilepsy patients. Among older individuals, there may be a higher prevalence of the disorder in females, although additional gender-related features are not clear and vary considerably with the gender distributions of the underlying medical conditions.

## Development and Course

Psychotic disorder due to another medical condition may be a single transient state or it may be recurrent, cycling with exacerbations and remissions of the underlying medical condition. Although treatment of the underlying medical condition often results in a resolution of the psychosis, this is not always the case, and psychotic symptoms may persist long after the medical event (e.g., psychotic disorder due to focal brain injury). In the context of chronic conditions such as multiple sclerosis or chronic interictal psychosis of epilepsy, the psychosis may assume a long-term course.

The expression of psychotic disorder due to another medical condition does not differ substantially in phenomenology depending on age at occurrence. However, older age groups have a higher prevalence of the disorder, which is most likely due to the increasing medical burden associated with advanced age and the cumulative effects of deleterious exposures and age-related processes (e.g., atherosclerosis). The nature of the underlying medical conditions is likely to change across the lifespan, with younger age groups more affected by epilepsy, head trauma, autoimmune, and neoplastic diseases of early to mid-life, and older age groups more affected by stroke disease, anoxic events, and multiple system comorbidities. Underlying factors with increasing age, such as preexisting cognitive impairment as well as vision and hearing impairments, may incur a greater risk for psychosis, possibly by serving to lower the threshold for experiencing psychosis.

# Risk and Prognostic Factors

**Course modifiers.**   Identification and treatment of the underlying medical condition has the greatest impact on course, although preexisting central nervous system injury may confer a worse course outcome (e.g., head trauma, cerebrovascular disease).

# Diagnostic Markers

The diagnosis of psychotic disorder due to another medical condition depends on the clinical condition of each individual, and the diagnostic tests will vary according to that condition. A variety of medical conditions may cause psychotic symptoms. These include neurological conditions (e.g., neoplasms, cerebrovascular disease, Huntington's disease, multiple sclerosis, epilepsy, auditory or visual nerve injury or impairment, deafness, migraine, central nervous system infections), endocrine conditions (e.g., hyper- and hypothyroidism, hyper- and hypoparathyroidism, hyper- and hypoadrenocorticism), metabolic conditions (e.g., hypoxia, hypercarbia, hypoglycemia), fluid or electrolyte imbalances, hepatic or renal diseases, and autoimmune disorders with central nervous system involvement (e.g., systemic lupus erythematosus). The associated physical examination findings, laboratory findings, and patterns of prevalence or onset reflect the etiological medical condition.

# Suicide Risk

Suicide risk in the context of psychotic disorder due to another medical condition is not clearly delineated, although certain conditions such as epilepsy and multiple sclerosis are associated with increased rates of suicide, which may be further increased in the presence of psychosis.

# Functional Consequences of Psychotic Disorder Due to Another Medical Condition

Functional disability is typically severe in the context of psychotic disorder due to another medical condition but will vary considerably by the type of condition and likely improve with successful resolution of the condition.

# Differential Diagnosis

**Delirium.**   Hallucinations and delusions commonly occur in the context of a delirium; however, a separate diagnosis of psychotic disorder due to another medical condition is not given if the disturbance occurs exclusively during the course of a delirium. Delusions in the context of a major or mild neurocognitive disorder would be diagnosed as major or mild neurocognitive disorder, with behavioral disturbance.

**Substance/medication-induced psychotic disorder.**   If there is evidence of recent or prolonged substance use (including medications with psychoactive effects), withdrawal from a substance, or exposure to a toxin (e.g., LSD [lysergic acid diethylamide] intoxication, alcohol withdrawal), a substance/medication-induced psychotic disorder should be considered. Symptoms that occur during or shortly after (i.e., within 4 weeks) of substance intoxication or withdrawal or after medication use may be especially indicative of a substance-induced psychotic disorder, depending on the character, duration, or amount of the substance used. If the clinician has ascertained that the disturbance is due to both a medical condition and substance use, both diagnoses (i.e., psychotic disorder due to another medical condition and substance/medication-induced psychotic disorder) can be given.

**Psychotic disorder.**   Psychotic disorder due to another medical condition must be distinguished from a psychotic disorder (e.g., schizophrenia, delusional disorder, schizoaffective disorder) or a depressive or bipolar disorder, with psychotic features. In psychotic disorders and in depressive or bipolar disorders, with psychotic features, no specific and direct causative physiological mechanisms associated with a medical condition can be demonstrated. Late age at onset and the absence of a personal or family history of schizophrenia or delusional disorder suggest the need for a thorough assessment to rule out the diagnosis of psychotic disorder due to another medical condition. Auditory hallucinations that involve voices speaking complex sentences are more characteristic of schizophrenia than of psychotic disorder due to a medical condition. Other types of hallucinations (e.g., visual, olfactory) commonly signal a psychotic disorder due to another medical condition or a substance/medication-induced psychotic disorder.

## Comorbidity

Psychotic disorder due to another medical condition in individuals older than 80 years is associated with concurrent major neurocognitive disorder (dementia).

# Catatonia

Catatonia can occur in the context of several disorders, including neurodevelopmental, psychotic, bipolar, depressive disorders, and other medical conditions (e.g., cerebral folate deficiency, rare autoimmune and paraneoplastic disorders. The manual does not treat catatonia as an independent class but recognizes a) catatonia associated with another mental disorder (i.e., a neurodevelopmental, psychotic disorder, a bipolar disorder, a depressive disorder, or other mental disorder), b) catatonic disorder due to another medical condition, and c) unspecified catatonia.

Catatonia is defined by the presence of three or more of 12 psychomotor features in the diagnostic criteria for catatonia associated with another mental disorder and catatonic disorder due to another medical condition. The essential feature of catatonia is a marked psychomotor disturbance that may involve decreased motor activity, decreased engagement during interview or physical examination, or excessive and peculiar motor activity. The clinical presentation of catatonia can be puzzling, as the psychomotor disturbance may range from marked unresponsiveness to marked agitation. Motoric immobility may be severe (stupor) or moderate (catalepsy and waxy flexibility). Similarly, decreased engagement may be severe (mutism) or moderate (negativism). Excessive and peculiar motor behaviors can be complex (e.g., stereotypy) or simple (agitation) and may include echolalia and echopraxia. In extreme cases, the same individual may wax and wane between decreased and excessive motor activity. The seemingly opposing clinical features and variable manifestations of the diagnosis contribute to a lack of awareness and decreased recognition of catatonia. During severe stages of catatonia, the individual may need careful supervision to avoid self-harm or harming others. There are potential risks from malnutrition, exhaustion, hyperpyrexia and self-inflicted injury.

# Catatonia Associated With Another Mental Disorder (Catatonia Specifier)

## 293.89 (F06.1)

A. The clinical picture is dominated by three (or more) of the following symptoms:

1. Stupor (i.e., no psychomotor activity; not actively relating to environment).
2. Catalepsy (i.e., passive induction of a posture held against gravity).
3. Waxy flexibility (i.e., slight, even resistance to positioning by examiner).
4. Mutism (i.e., no, or very little, verbal response [exclude if known aphasia]).
5. Negativism (i.e., opposition or no response to instructions or external stimuli).
6. Posturing (i.e., spontaneous and active maintenance of a posture against gravity).
7. Mannerism (i.e., odd, circumstantial caricature of normal actions).
8. Stereotypy (i.e., repetitive, abnormally frequent, non-goal-directed movements).
9. Agitation, not influenced by external stimuli.
10. Grimacing.
11. Echolalia (i.e., mimicking another's speech).
12. Echopraxia (i.e., mimicking another's movements).

**Coding note:** Indicate the name of the associated mental disorder when recording the name of the condition (i.e., 293.89 [F06.1] catatonia associated with major depressive disorder). Code first the associated mental disorder (e.g., neurodevelopmental disorder, brief psychotic disorder, schizophreniform disorder, schizophrenia, schizoaffective disorder, bipolar disorder, major depressive disorder, or other mental disorder) (e.g., 295.70 [F25.1] schizoaffective disorder, depressive type; 293.89 [F06.1] catatonia associated with schizoaffective disorder).

## Diagnostic Features

Catatonia associated with another mental disorder (catatonia specifier) may be used when criteria are met for catatonia during the course of a neurodevelopmental, psychotic, bipolar, depressive, or other mental disorder. The catatonia specifier is appropriate when the clinical picture is characterized by marked psychomotor disturbance and involves at least three of the 12 diagnostic features listed in Criterion A. Catatonia is typically diagnosed in an inpatient setting and occurs in up to 35% of individuals with schizophrenia, but the majority of catatonia cases involve individuals with depressive or bipolar disorders. Before the catatonia specifier is used in neurodevelopmental, psychotic, bipolar, depressive, or other mental disorders, a wide variety of other medical conditions need to be ruled out; these conditions include, but are not limited to, medical conditions due to infectious, metabolic, or neurological conditions (see "Catatonic Disorder Due to Another Medical Condition"). Catatonia can also be a side effect of a medication (see the DSM-5 chapter "Medication-Induced Movement Disorders and Other Adverse Effects of Medication"). Because of the seriousness of the complications, particular attention should be paid to the possibility that the catatonia is attributable to 333.92 (G21.0) neuroleptic malignant syndrome.

# Catatonic Disorder Due to Another Medical Condition

## Diagnostic Criteria                                   293.89 (F06.1)

A. The clinical picture is dominated by three (or more) of the following symptoms:
    1. Stupor (i.e., no psychomotor activity; not actively relating to environment).
    2. Catalepsy (i.e., passive induction of a posture held against gravity).
    3. Waxy flexibility (i.e., slight, even resistance to positioning by examiner).
    4. Mutism (i.e., no, or very little, verbal response [**Note:** not applicable if there is an established aphasia]).
    5. Negativism (i.e., opposition or no response to instructions or external stimuli).
    6. Posturing (i.e., spontaneous and active maintenance of a posture against gravity).
    7. Mannerism (i.e., odd, circumstantial caricature of normal actions).
    8. Stereotypy (i.e., repetitive, abnormally frequent, non-goal-directed movements).
    9. Agitation, not influenced by external stimuli.
    10. Grimacing.
    11. Echolalia (i.e., mimicking another's speech).
    12. Echopraxia (i.e., mimicking another's movements).

B. There is evidence from the history, physical examination, or laboratory findings that the disturbance is the direct pathophysiological consequence of another medical condition.

C. The disturbance is not better explained by another mental disorder (e.g., a manic episode).

D. The disturbance does not occur exclusively during the course of a delirium.

E. The disturbance causes clinically significant distress or impairment in social, occupational, or other important areas of functioning.

**Coding note:** Include the name of the medical condition in the name of the mental disorder (e.g., 293.89 [F06.1]) catatonic disorder due to hepatic encephalopathy). The other medical condition should be coded and listed separately immediately before the catatonic disorder due to the medical condition (e.g., 572.2 [K71.90] hepatic encephalopathy; 293.89 [F06.1] catatonic disorder due to hepatic encephalopathy).

## Diagnostic Features

The essential feature of catatonic disorder due to another medical condition is the presence of catatonia that is judged to be attributed to the physiological effects of another medical condition. Catatonia can be diagnosed by the presence of at least three of the 12 clinical features in Criterion A. There must be evidence from the history, physical examination, or laboratory findings that the catatonia is attributable to another medical condition (Criterion B). The diagnosis is not given if the catatonia is better explained by another mental disorder (e.g., manic episode) (Criterion C) or if it occurs exclusively during the course of a delirium (Criterion D).

## Associated Features Supporting Diagnosis

A variety of medical conditions may cause catatonia, especially neurological conditions (e.g., neoplasms, head trauma, cerebrovascular disease, encephalitis) and metabolic conditions (e.g., hypercalcemia, hepatic encephalopathy, homocystinuria, diabetic ketoacidosis). The associated physical examination findings, laboratory findings, and patterns of prevalence and onset reflect those of the etiological medical condition.

## Differential Diagnosis

A separate diagnosis of catatonic disorder due to another medical condition is not given if the catatonia occurs exclusively during the course of a delirium or neuroleptic malignant syndrome. If the individual is currently taking neuroleptic medication, consideration should be given to medication-induced movement disorders (e.g., abnormal positioning may be due to neuroleptic-induced acute dystonia) or neuroleptic malignant syndrome (e.g., catatonic-like features may be present, along with associated vital sign and/or laboratory abnormalities). Catatonic symptoms may be present in any of the following five psychotic disorders: brief psychotic disorder, schizophreniform disorder, schizophrenia, schizoaffective disorder, and substance/medication-induced psychotic disorder. It may also be present in some of the neurodevelopmental disorders, in all of the bipolar and depressive disorders, and in other mental disorders.

# Unspecified Catatonia

This category applies to presentations in which symptoms characteristic of catatonia cause clinically significant distress or impairment in social, occupational, or other important areas of functioning but either the nature of the underlying mental disorder or other medical condition is unclear, full criteria for catatonia are not met, or there is insufficient information to make a more specific diagnosis (e.g., in emergency room settings).

**Coding note:** Code first **781.99 (R29.818)** other symptoms involving nervous and musculoskeletal systems, followed by **293.89 (F06.1)** unspecified catatonia.

# Other Specified Schizophrenia Spectrum and Other Psychotic Disorder

## 298.8 (F28)

This category applies to presentations in which symptoms characteristic of a schizophrenia spectrum and other psychotic disorder that cause clinically significant distress or impairment in social, occupational, or other important areas of functioning predominate but do not meet the full criteria for any of the disorders in the schizophrenia spectrum and other psychotic disorders diagnostic class. The other specified schizophrenia spectrum and other psychotic disorder category is used in situations in which the clinician chooses to communicate the specific reason that the presentation does not meet the criteria for any specific schizophrenia spectrum and other psychotic disorder. This is done by recording "other specified schizophrenia spectrum and other psychotic disorder" followed by the specific reason (e.g., "persistent auditory hallucinations").

Examples of presentations that can be specified using the "other specified" designation include the following:

1. **Persistent auditory hallucinations** occurring in the absence of any other features.
2. **Delusions with significant overlapping mood episodes:** This includes persistent delusions with periods of overlapping mood episodes that are present for a substantial portion of the delusional disturbance (such that the criterion stipulating only brief mood disturbance in delusional disorder is not met).
3. **Attenuated psychosis syndrome:** This syndrome is characterized by psychotic-like symptoms that are below a threshold for full psychosis (e.g., the symptoms are less severe and more transient, and insight is relatively maintained).
4. **Delusional symptoms in partner of individual with delusional disorder:** In the context of a relationship, the delusional material from the dominant partner provides content for delusional belief by the individual who may not otherwise entirely meet criteria for delusional disorder.

# Unspecified Schizophrenia Spectrum and Other Psychotic Disorder

## 298.9 (F29)

This category applies to presentations in which symptoms characteristic of a schizophrenia spectrum and other psychotic disorder that cause clinically significant distress or impairment in social, occupational, or other important areas of functioning predominate but do not meet the full criteria for any of the disorders in the schizophrenia spectrum and other psychotic disorders diagnostic class. The unspecified schizophrenia spectrum and other psychotic disorder category is used in situations in which the clinician chooses *not* to specify the reason that the criteria are not met for a specific schizophrenia spectrum and other psychotic disorder, and includes presentations in which there is insufficient information to make a more specific diagnosis (e.g., in emergency room settings).

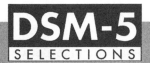

# Schizophrenia Spectrum and Other Psychotic Disorders

## DSM-5® Guidebook

| | |
|---|---|
| **301.22 (F21)** | Schizotypal (Personality) Disorder (see also "Personality Disorders") |
| **297.1 (F22)** | Delusional Disorder |
| **298.8 (F23)** | Brief Psychotic Disorder |
| **295.40 (F20.81)** | Schizophreniform Disorder |
| **295.90 (F20.9)** | Schizophrenia |
| **295.70 (F25._)** | Schizoaffective Disorder |
| | Substance/Medication-Induced Psychotic Disorder |
| | Psychotic Disorder Due to Another Medical Condition |
| **293.89 (F06.1)** | Catatonia Associated With Another Mental Disorder (Catatonia Specifier) |
| **293.89 (F06.1)** | Catatonic Disorder Due to Another Medical Condition |
| **293.89 (F06.1)** | Unspecified Catatonia |
| **298.8 (F28)** | Other Specified Schizophrenia Spectrum and Other Psychotic Disorder |
| **298.9 (F29)** | Unspecified Schizophrenia Spectrum and Other Psychotic Disorder |

The diagnostic class schizophrenia spectrum and other psychotic disorders comprises schizophrenia and related disorders, other major psychoses, and disorders with subthreshold psychoses (Table 1). All are unified by the presence of one or more of the following five domains of psychopathology: delusions, hallucinations, disorganized thinking, grossly disorganized or catatonic behavior, and negative symptoms. Whereas the first four domains are examples of psychosis, negative symptoms are characterized by the absence of something that should be present, such as fluency and spontaneity of verbal expression. The term *psychosis* holds different meanings, but beginning with DSM-III, the term has had a more restricted definition that requires the person to experience a break with reality. In the psychoanalytic era, the term was often used to describe persons who were severely ill and functionally impaired but had a broad range of problems and symptoms.

Schizophrenia is arguably the most disabling of the psychoses, yet other psychotic disorders are also important to recognize and diagnose. These include delusional disorder, brief psychotic disorder, schizophreniform disorder, and schizoaffective disorder. The chapter also includes psychoses that are attributable to other medical conditions or are induced by substances or medications. Catatonic disorder due to another med-

TABLE 1.   DSM-5 schizophrenia spectrum and other psychotic disorders

Schizotypal (personality) disorder (see Chapter 18, "Personality Disorders" [in DSM-5])

Delusional disorder

Brief psychotic disorder

Schizophreniform disorder

Schizophrenia

Schizoaffective disorder

Substance/medication-induced psychotic disorder

Psychotic disorder due to another medical condition

Catatonia associated with another mental disorder (catatonia specifier)

Catatonic disorder due to another medical condition

Unspecified catatonia

Other specified schizophrenia spectrum and other psychotic disorder

Unspecified schizophrenia spectrum and other psychotic disorder

ical condition has been moved to this chapter and is used for those cases in which the disorder is medically induced. Unspecified catatonia is new to DSM-5. Other specified and unspecified schizophrenia spectrum and other psychotic disorders constitute residual categories that are used to describe psychotic symptoms that do not fit into any of the better-defined categories.

All psychotic disorders are included in this chapter of DSM-5 except those related to bipolar disorder, depressive disorders, or a neurocognitive disorder. This organization should help facilitate the differential diagnosis of psychotic disorders.

Several important changes have been made to this class. The most basic change involves overall chapter organization. Disorders are now arranged along a gradient from least to most severe. Severity is defined by the level, number, and duration of psychotic signs and symptoms. DSM-5 cautions users to diagnose more severe conditions once the lesser conditions are ruled out. Clinicians know (and trainees learn) that for many individuals the diagnostic process may take months or even years because signs and symptoms evolve gradually. For example, a young man evaluated for social withdrawal and magical thinking may have symptoms that initially meet criteria for schizotypal personality disorder, but several years later he may develop frank delusions and hallucinations that meet criteria for schizophrenia. At the same time, the clinician needs to have ruled out alternative explanations, such as a substance use disorder or another medical condition, in order to arrive at the best diagnosis.

Schizotypal personality disorder is included in this chapter because of its membership in the schizophrenia spectrum, but criteria and text are found with the personality disorders (see chapter "Personality Disorders" in DSM-5). The criteria for delusional disorder are mostly unchanged, but the adjective *nonbizarre* has been removed (Criterion A), and the somatic subtype has been edited to ensure that those who are delusional regarding a "physical defect" are more appropriately diagnosed with body dysmorphic disorder, now placed in the DSM-5 chapter "Obsessive-Compulsive and

Related Disorders." In DSM-IV, body dysmorphic disorder was included with the somatoform disorders.

Shared psychotic disorder has been eliminated because the diagnosis was infrequently used and persons whose symptoms met criteria for the diagnosis generally also met criteria for some other psychotic disorder (e.g., delusional disorder). The essence of shared psychotic disorder is the transmission of delusional beliefs from one person to another. In the past, these rare cases were called *folie à deux*, a French term for "double insanity."

Clinicians will no longer record schizophrenia subtypes. Although the paranoid, disorganized, catatonic, undifferentiated, and residual subtypes have a lengthy history that predates DSM-I (McGlashan and Fenton 1994), there was little evidence to support either their clinical utility or their predictive validity (Helmes and Landmark 2003). Because the course of schizophrenia is highly variable, the subtypes had little stability, so that at various stages of illness it was not unusual for a person's symptoms to meet criteria for different subtypes. For example, a person's symptoms may have met the criteria for disorganized subtype early in the illness and then met criteria for the paranoid subtype and, eventually, the residual subtype later in the course of the illness.

The criteria for schizoaffective disorder have been modified to provide more guidance to clinicians regarding the total duration of mood symptoms. Instead of requiring that mood symptoms last a "substantial portion of the total duration of the active and residual periods of the illness" (as in DSM-IV [American Psychiatric Association 1994]), DSM-5 requires that they be present for a "majority of the total duration of the active and residual portions of the illness." The change was prompted by the low reliability of the criterion and its limited clinical utility.

The Psychotic Disorders Work Group had debated the possible inclusion of attenuated psychosis syndrome. The syndrome is a collection of symptoms associated with a high probability of the person developing schizophrenia. The impetus to include this condition was that it would help to identify those likely to develop schizophrenia, thereby allowing early clinical attention and treatment. The decision was made to include this syndrome in Section III, in "Conditions for Further Study" (see Chapter 22) but include it as an example of an other specified schizophrenia spectrum and other psychotic disorder.

# Schizotypal (Personality) Disorder

Schizotypal personality disorder is included in this chapter because of its presence within the schizophrenia specturum. Criteria and text for the disorder are found in the DSM-5 chapter on personality disorders.

# Delusional Disorder

Delusional disorder is a diagnosis used in individuals who have persistent delusions but relatively normal psychosocial functioning apart from the ramifications of the delusions and who exhibit behavior that is not obviously odd or bizarre. First included in DSM-III under the rubric "paranoid disorder," the name was changed to delusional (paranoid) disorder in DSM-III-R because while delusions are the primary symptoms, the term *paranoid* has many other meanings.

Delusional disorders have a long history. Kraepelin distinguished paranoia from *dementia praecox* and used the diagnosis for persons with systematized delusions (but no hallucinations) and a prolonged course without recovery but not leading to mental deterioration. Traditionally, the diagnosis has been used for persons who have non-bizarre (i.e., possible but not plausible) delusions but whose functioning is relatively well preserved, without the deterioration in functioning seen in persons with schizophrenia and schizoaffective disorder. Because these individuals experience their delusional beliefs as ego-syntonic (i.e., consistent with their own expectations, sense of self, and sense of reality in general), their insight is poor and they generally have little interest in seeking treatment.

In DSM-5, a number of changes have been made to the diagnosis. The adjective *nonbizarre* has been removed from Criterion A. One reason is that "bizarreness" is often hard to judge, especially across different cultures (Cermolacce et al. 2010). Another reason behind the change is more practical and stems in part from a change in the definition of schizophrenia, in which the special treatment of bizarre delusions has been deleted from Criterion A. With this change, the presence of a single bizarre delusion no longer satisfies Criterion A for schizophrenia. Removing the term *nonbizarre* from the criteria for delusional disorder was necessary to allow a place within the delusional disorder category for the rare individual with a single bizarre delusion. The work group found little justification for differential treatment of delusions based on whether they are bizarre or nonbizarre. The addition of the "with bizarre content" specifier allows for the recording of the nature of the delusion and permits continuity with DSM-IV. This specifier is used when the delusions are thought to be clearly implausible.

Criterion E has been added to rule out other mental disorders, including body dysmorphic disorder and obsessive-compulsive disorder. In addition, the somatic subtype has been edited to delete the phrase "some physical defect." Both changes will help ensure that those who are delusional regarding a "physical defect" are more appropriately diagnosed with body dysmorphic disorder, which is now included with the new diagnostic class obsessive-compulsive and related disorders (see Chapter 7). The work group felt that this change was necessary because people with body dysmorphic disorder—delusional or not—have a course of illness similar to those with obsessive-compulsive disorder, and tend to respond to selective serotonin reuptake inhibitor medications. The changes help to distinguish delusional disorder from body dysmorphic disorder, with absent insight/delusional beliefs, and obsessive-compulsive disorder, with absent insight/delusional beliefs.

---

## Diagnostic Criteria for Delusional Disorder    **297.1 (F22)**

---

A. The presence of one (or more) delusions with a duration of 1 month or longer.
B. Criterion A for schizophrenia has never been met.
   **Note:** Hallucinations, if present, are not prominent and are related to the delusional theme (e.g., the sensation of being infested with insects associated with delusions of infestation).

C. Apart from the impact of the delusion(s) or its ramifications, functioning is not markedly impaired, and behavior is not obviously bizarre or odd.

D. If manic or major depressive episodes have occurred, these have been brief relative to the duration of the delusional periods.

E. The disturbance is not attributable to the physiological effects of a substance or another medical condition and is not better explained by another mental disorder, such as body dysmorphic disorder or obsessive-compulsive disorder.

*Specify* whether:

**Erotomanic type:** This subtype applies when the central theme of the delusion is that another person is in love with the individual.

**Grandiose type:** This subtype applies when the central theme of the delusion is the conviction of having some great (but unrecognized) talent or insight or having made some important discovery.

**Jealous type:** This subtype applies when the central theme of the individual's delusion is that his or her spouse or lover is unfaithful.

**Persecutory type:** This subtype applies when the central theme of the delusion involves the individual's belief that he or she is being conspired against, cheated, spied on, followed, poisoned or drugged, maliciously maligned, harassed, or obstructed in the pursuit of long-term goals.

**Somatic type:** This subtype applies when the central theme of the delusion involves bodily functions or sensations.

**Mixed type:** This subtype applies when no one delusional theme predominates.

**Unspecified type:** This subtype applies when the dominant delusional belief cannot be clearly determined or is not described in the specific types (e.g., referential delusions without a prominent persecutory or grandiose component).

*Specify* if:

**With bizarre content:** Delusions are deemed bizarre if they are clearly implausible, not understandable, and not derived from ordinary life experiences (e.g., an individual's belief that a stranger has removed his or her internal organs and replaced them with someone else's organs without leaving any wounds or scars).

*Specify* if:

The following course specifiers are only to be used after a 1-year duration of the disorder:

**First episode, currently in acute episode:** First manifestation of the disorder meeting the defining diagnostic symptom and time criteria. An *acute episode* is a time period in which the symptom criteria are fulfilled.

**First episode, currently in partial remission:** *Partial remission* is a time period during which an improvement after a previous episode is maintained and in which the defining criteria of the disorder are only partially fulfilled.

**First episode, currently in full remission:** *Full remission* is a period of time after a previous episode during which no disorder-specific symptoms are present.

**Multiple episodes, currently in acute episode**

**Multiple episodes, currently in partial remission**

**Multiple episodes, currently in full remission**

**Continuous:** Symptoms fulfilling the diagnostic symptom criteria of the disorder are remaining for the majority of the illness course, with subthreshold symptom periods being very brief relative to the overall course.

**Unspecified**

*Specify* current severity:

Severity is rated by a quantitative assessment of the primary symptoms of psychosis, including delusions, hallucinations, disorganized speech, abnormal psychomotor behavior, and negative symptoms. Each of these symptoms may be rated for its current severity (most severe in the last 7 days) on a 5-point scale ranging from 0 (not present) to 4 (present and severe). (See Clinician-Rated Dimensions of Psychosis Symptom Severity in Chapter 20, "Assessment Measures," this volume.)
**Note:** Diagnosis of delusional disorder can be made without using this severity specifier.

## Criterion A

Delusional disorder requires the presence of delusions for a minimum of 1 month. DSM-IV specified that the delusions were nonbizarre. Although the term *nonbizarre* has been deleted, the spirit of the disorder as involving persons with nonbizarre delusions remains, as indicated by the various subtypes. Individuals with schizophrenia often have very bizarre delusions not possible in real life. For example, we have had patients claim they are being controlled by radio transmitters implanted in their brains (although with rapidly developing technology, that situation may be possible in the future).

## Criterion B

Excluding symptoms that meet Criterion A of schizophrenia has helped to separate delusional disorder from schizophrenia. People with schizophrenia have other psychotic symptoms (hallucinations; disorganized speech; grossly abnormal behavior, including catatonia) in addition to negative symptoms. Although individuals with delusional disorder may have tactile and olfactory hallucinations that relate to their delusion, they are otherwise free of those symptoms common to persons with schizophrenia (e.g., auditory hallucinations). For example, individuals with delusional disorder, somatic type, may have delusions of being infested with parasites and report feeling them moving about under their skin. (This particular delusion has been referred to as *delusional parasitosis* and is more commonly seen by dermatologists.)

## Criterion C

People with delusional disorder do not behave in an obviously odd or bizarre fashion. This is an important distinction from people with schizophrenia, who often act in strange ways, such as muttering to themselves, wearing dirty or inappropriate clothing, or accosting strangers. The purpose of this criterion is to ensure that delusional disorder is restricted to persons who, apart from their delusion or its ramifications, are able to function. That said, the behavior of some persons is greatly influenced by their delusions, and this can be reflected in their actions. For example, a person in love with a television actress may attempt to contact the person, or in rare cases may stalk her. A person who thinks his wife is unfaithful may read her private e-mail or monitor her daily activities in an attempt to catch her with the paramour.

## Criterion D

If persons with delusional disorder have had concurrent mood episodes, these episodes must have been relatively brief. The goal is to separate delusional disorder from psychotic forms of major depressive disorder. Individuals with the latter may develop delusions in the context of suffering severe depression, but these delusions tend to have depressive content, such as believing oneself to have committed a sinful act or to have lost all of one's savings. If the delusions occur exclusively during the course of the depressive illness, the diagnosis is a mood disorder with psychotic features.

Individuals with delusional disorder often have significant depressive symptoms. The clinician may feel that the symptoms merit an independent diagnosis of major depressive disorder or other specified or unspecified depressive disorder (or if there is a bipolar course, other specified or unspecified bipolar and related disorder). Schizoaffective disorder is another diagnostic possibility if the delusions are long-standing and the mood disorder is severe.

## Criterion E

This criterion excludes delusional disorders attributable to the physiological effects of a substance or another medical condition or are better explained by another mental disorder. Delusions can result from a variety of medical illnesses, certain medical treatments or medications (e.g., corticosteroids), and use of drugs of abuse (e.g., stimulants). This criterion requires ruling out neurocognitive disorders, such as a dementia, as well as traumatic brain injuries or a convulsive disorder. Also, certain forms of body dysmorphic disorder and obsessive-compulsive disorder are relatively severe and are associated with delusions (e.g., when an individual believes his normal-appearing nose is ugly and misshapen). Even when the belief reaches delusional proportions, the diagnosis body dysmorphic disorder is more appropriate than delusional disorder.

## Subtypes and Specifiers

Subtypes are used to indicate the specific theme the disorder has taken, such as erotomania or grandiosity. Bizarreness, course of the disorder, and current severity can also be specified.

# Brief Psychotic Disorder

Brief psychotic disorder is a diagnosis used for relatively brief episodes of psychosis lasting at least 1 day but less than 1 month. The disorder is relatively uncommon and occurs in persons who otherwise have not experienced a decline in their day-to-day functioning or who display signs that in retrospect suggest the prodrome of schizophrenia. Further, the psychotic symptoms associated with this diagnosis tend to be brought on by stressful situations or acute mood changes. In the past, this diagnosis was often referred to as a reactive, hysterical, or psychogenic psychosis. The diagnosis is essentially unchanged from DSM-IV except for minor editing and the addition of the specifiers for catatonia and current severity.

Some individuals report new-onset psychotic symptoms that last minutes to hours and that therefore do not qualify for the diagnosis. These symptoms can occur in persons with borderline personality disorder or schizotypal personality disorder; in these cases no additional diagnosis is necessary. Otherwise, when these short-lived symptoms occur, and they are not attributable to a medication, a drug of abuse, or another medical condition, the diagnosis other specified or unspecified schizophrenia spectrum and other psychotic disorder may be appropriate.

---

## Diagnostic Criteria for Brief Psychotic Disorder          **298.8 (F23)**

---

A. Presence of one (or more) of the following symptoms. At least one of these must be (1), (2), or (3):

 1. Delusions.
 2. Hallucinations.
 3. Disorganized speech (e.g., frequent derailment or incoherence).
 4. Grossly disorganized or catatonic behavior.
 **Note:** Do not include a symptom if it is a culturally sanctioned response.
B. Duration of an episode of the disturbance is at least 1 day but less than 1 month, with eventual full return to premorbid level of functioning.
C. The disturbance is not better explained by major depressive or bipolar disorder with psychotic features or another psychotic disorder such as schizophrenia or catatonia, and is not attributable to the physiological effects of a substance (e.g., a drug of abuse, a medication) or another medical condition.

*Specify* if:
 **With marked stressor(s)** (brief reactive psychosis): If symptoms occur in response to events that, singly or together, would be markedly stressful to almost anyone in similar circumstances in the individual's culture.
 **Without marked stressor(s):** If symptoms do not occur in response to events that, singly or together, would be markedly stressful to almost anyone in similar circumstances in the individual's culture.
 **With postpartum onset:** If onset is during pregnancy or within 4 weeks postpartum.

*Specify* if:
 **With catatonia** (refer to the criteria for catatonia associated with another mental disorder, [DSM-5] pp. 119–120, for definition)
   **Coding note:** Use additional code 293.89 (F06.1) catatonia associated with brief psychotic disorder to indicate the presence of the comorbid catatonia.

*Specify* current severity:
 Severity is rated by a quantitative assessment of the primary symptoms of psychosis, including delusions, hallucinations, disorganized speech, abnormal psychomotor behavior, and negative symptoms. Each of these symptoms may be rated for its current severity (most severe in the last 7 days) on a 5-point scale ranging from 0 (not present) to 4 (present and severe). (See Clinician-Rated Dimensions of Psychosis Symptom Severity in the chapter "Assessment Measures" [in DSM-5].)
 **Note:** Diagnosis of brief psychotic disorder can be made without using this severity specifier.

---

## Criterion A

Psychotic symptoms must be present, and the Criterion A list for brief psychotic disorder replicates that for schizophrenia *except* that negative symptoms are not included; these usually occur over long periods of time and do not generally present acutely. The diagnosis does not apply when the psychotic symptoms appear to have developed in response to culturally sanctioned activities, such as *Qigong*, a Chinese health-enhancing practice that can reportedly lead to transient psychosis. This is an important consideration, because psychotic-like phenomena are reported to occur during extended religious or ceremonial rituals in several non-Western cultures.

## Criterion B

The disturbance lasts at least 1 day but less than 1 month. If the duration is longer, the person will presumably qualify for another diagnosis, such as schizophreniform disorder.

## Criterion C

The language has been edited for consistency within DSM-5, but otherwise this criterion is unchanged from DSM-IV. Mood disorders, other psychotic disorders, medical conditions, and the physiological effects of substances need to be ruled out as a cause of the disturbance.

## Specifiers

When the disorder occurs in response to stressors, the clinician can use the specifier "with marked stressor(s)." If brief psychotic disorder occurs within 4 weeks postpartum, the "with postpartum onset" specifier is appropriate. Typically, women with postpartum onset generally develop symptoms within 1–2 weeks of delivery. Symptoms can include disorganized speech, misperceptions, labile mood, confusion, and hallucinations. Frequently referred to as "postpartum psychosis," the disorder tends to arise in otherwise normally functioning individuals. The disorder should be distinguished from the "baby blues," which occurs in many new mothers and may last for a few days after delivery but is not considered pathologic. The new specifier "with catatonia" can be used when the full syndrome is present. Current severity can be specified as well.

# Schizophreniform Disorder

The term *schizophreniform* was used by Gabriel Langfeldt (1939) to describe acute psychoses that were reactive and occurred in persons with relatively normal personalities. Such cases were referred to as "acute schizophrenic episodes" in DSM-II. Schizophreniform disorder was formally recognized in DSM-III as one of several psychotic disorders not elsewhere classified. The diagnosis is used for symptoms of schizophrenia that last at least 1 month but less than 6 months. Once the symptoms have lasted 6 months or longer, the diagnosis changes to schizophrenia, even if only residual symptoms remain (e.g., blunted affect).

The validity of schizophreniform disorder has been debated. Some individuals diagnosed with this disorder develop schizophrenia, whereas others develop a mood disorder or schizoaffective disorder. Persons with schizophreniform disorder have a relatively better prognosis than those diagnosed with schizophrenia at first encounter.

---

## Diagnostic Criteria for Schizophreniform Disorder    295.40 (F20.81)

---

A. Two (or more) of the following, each present for a significant portion of time during a 1-month period (or less if successfully treated). At least one of these must be (1), (2), or (3):

   1. Delusions.
   2. Hallucinations.
   3. Disorganized speech (e.g., frequent derailment or incoherence).
   4. Grossly disorganized or catatonic behavior.
   5. Negative symptoms (i.e., diminished emotional expression or avolition).

B. An episode of the disorder lasts at least 1 month but less than 6 months. When the diagnosis must be made without waiting for recovery, it should be qualified as "provisional."

C. Schizoaffective disorder and depressive or bipolar disorder with psychotic features have been ruled out because either 1) no major depressive or manic episodes have occurred concurrently with the active-phase symptoms, or 2) if mood episodes have occurred during active-phase symptoms, they have been present for a minority of the total duration of the active and residual periods of the illness.

D. The disturbance is not attributable to the physiological effects of a substance (e.g., a drug of abuse, a medication) or another medical condition.

*Specify* if:

**With good prognostic features:** This specifier requires the presence of at least two of the following features: onset of prominent psychotic symptoms within 4 weeks of the first noticeable change in usual behavior or functioning; confusion or perplexity; good premorbid social and occupational functioning; and absence of blunted or flat affect.

**Without good prognostic features:** This specifier is applied if two or more of the above features have not been present.

*Specify* if:

**With catatonia** (refer to the criteria for catatonia associated with another mental disorder, [DSM-5] pp. 119–120, for definition).

   **Coding note:** Use additional code 293.89 (F06.1) catatonia associated with schizophreniform disorder to indicate the presence of the comorbid catatonia.

*Specify* current severity:

Severity is rated by a quantitative assessment of the primary symptoms of psychosis, including delusions, hallucinations, disorganized speech, abnormal psychomotor behavior, and negative symptoms. Each of these symptoms may be rated for its current severity (most severe in the last 7 days) on a 5-point scale ranging from 0 (not present) to 4 (present and severe). (See Clinician-Rated Dimensions of Psychosis Symptom Severity in the chapter "Assessment Measures" [in DSM-5].) **Note:** Diagnosis of schizophreniform disorder can be made without using this severity specifier.

---

The criteria require that the individual's symptoms meet schizophrenia Criterion A (psychotic symptoms), as well as schizophrenia Criteria D and E (which require that other mental disorders, substances of abuse, and other medical disorders have been ruled out as a cause of the disorder). Because the individual would have new-onset symptoms, alternative explanations need to be ruled out during a comprehensive evaluation.

The clinician should specify whether the individual has good prognostic features, such as acute onset, confusion or perplexity, good premorbid functioning, and absence of a flattened affect—all of which are symptoms identified in research studies as correlating with good prognosis. Catatonic features should be specified if present. Current severity can also be specified.

# Schizophrenia

In DSM-5, schizophrenia is defined by a group of characteristic symptoms, such as delusions, hallucinations, and negative symptoms (i.e., diminished emotional expression or avolition); deterioration in social, occupational, or interpersonal functioning; and continuous signs of the disturbance for at least 6 months. No symptoms are specific—or pathognomonic—to schizophrenia, complicating the task of establishing the proper boundaries for the disorder.

Kraepelin (1919) is generally credited for producing the first coherent definition of schizophrenia, which he called *dementia praecox*. His conceptualization was of an early onset illness characterized by psychotic symptoms with a chronic and deteriorating course. He was also instrumental in separating dementia praecox from manic-depressive illness, which had its onset throughout life and had a more episodic course. Kraepelin's emphasis on psychotic symptoms and a deteriorating course helped to identify a relatively narrow group of severely ill patients with chronic symptoms and poor prognosis.

*Dementia praecox* was eventually renamed *schizophrenia* by Bleuler (1950) in 1911 to emphasize the cognitive impairment that occurs, which he saw as a "splitting" of the psychic processes. Bleuler maintained that certain symptoms were fundamental to the illness, including affective blunting, disturbance of association (i.e., peculiar and distorted thinking), autism, and indecisiveness (ambivalence). He de-emphasized course and regarded delusions and hallucinations as accessory symptoms because they could occur in other disorders. Bleuler's ideas earned acceptance and guided the practice of generations of American and European psychiatrists who were taught the importance of Bleuler's fundamental symptoms ("the four A's"). Because these symptoms were imprecise, they defined a much more heterogeneous group of patients, often much less ill than those identified by Kraepelin, and contributed to an increasingly broad concept of schizophrenia.

The ideas of Kurt Schneider (1959) helped reshape the concept of schizophrenia into that of a relatively severe psychotic disorder, bringing it back to the original ideas of Kraepelin. He described "first-rank" psychotic symptoms that he believed were relatively specific and that thus helped to discriminate schizophrenia from other disorders. These symptoms included thought insertion, thought withdrawal, thought broadcasting, voices communicating with (or about) the person, and delusions of being externally controlled (i.e., delusions of passivity). Schneider's description of schizophrenia emphasized the presence of one or more of these psychotic symptoms and was cross-sectional in its definition of the illness. Although later research suggested that these "Schneiderian" symptoms were not particularly specific (Nordgaard et al. 2008), Schneider's ideas gained prominence and influenced DSM-III, DSM-III-R, and DSM-IV with their special treatment of "bizarre" delusions and certain hallucinations.

With DSM-5, modest changes have been made in the criteria for schizophrenia. The main change has been to eliminate the special status of Schneiderian first-rank symptoms, including bizarre delusions and certain hallucinations such as voices conversing. The recommendation was also made to eliminate schizophrenia subtypes. Work group members agreed that the classic subtypes provided a poor description of the heterogeneity of the disorder and had low diagnostic stability, with only the paranoid and undifferentiated subtypes being used with any frequency.

---

## Diagnostic Criteria for Schizophrenia                   **295.90 (F20.9)**

---

A. Two (or more) of the following, each present for a significant portion of time during a 1-month period (or less if successfully treated). At least one of these must be (1), (2), or (3):

1. Delusions.
2. Hallucinations.
3. Disorganized speech (e.g., frequent derailment or incoherence).
4. Grossly disorganized or catatonic behavior.
5. Negative symptoms (i.e., diminished emotional expression or avolition).

B. For a significant portion of the time since the onset of the disturbance, level of functioning in one or more major areas, such as work, interpersonal relations, or self-care, is markedly below the level achieved prior to the onset (or when the onset is in childhood or adolescence, there is failure to achieve expected level of interpersonal, academic, or occupational functioning).

C. Continuous signs of the disturbance persist for at least 6 months. This 6-month period must include at least 1 month of symptoms (or less if successfully treated) that meet Criterion A (i.e., active-phase symptoms) and may include periods of prodromal or residual symptoms. During these prodromal or residual periods, the signs of the disturbance may be manifested by only negative symptoms or by two or more symptoms listed in Criterion A present in an attenuated form (e.g., odd beliefs, unusual perceptual experiences).

D. Schizoaffective disorder and depressive or bipolar disorder with psychotic features have been ruled out because either 1) no major depressive or manic episodes have occurred concurrently with the active-phase symptoms, or 2) if mood episodes have occurred during active-phase symptoms, they have been present for a minority of the total duration of the active and residual periods of the illness.

E. The disturbance is not attributable to the physiological effects of a substance (e.g., a drug of abuse, a medication) or another medical condition.

F. If there is a history of autism spectrum disorder or a communication disorder of childhood onset, the additional diagnosis of schizophrenia is made only if prominent delusions or hallucinations, in addition to the other required symptoms of schizophrenia, are also present for at least 1 month (or less if successfully treated).

*Specify* if:

The following course specifiers are only to be used after a 1-year duration of the disorder and if they are not in contradiction to the diagnostic course criteria.

**First episode, currently in acute episode:** First manifestation of the disorder meeting the defining diagnostic symptom and time criteria. An *acute episode* is a time period in which the symptom criteria are fulfilled.

**First episode, currently in partial remission:** *Partial remission* is a period of time during which an improvement after a previous episode is maintained and in which the defining criteria of the disorder are only partially fulfilled.

**First episode, currently in full remission:** *Full remission* is a period of time after a previous episode during which no disorder-specific symptoms are present.

**Multiple episodes, currently in acute episode:** Multiple episodes may be determined after a minimum of two episodes (i.e., after a first episode, a remission and a minimum of one relapse).

**Multiple episodes, currently in partial remission**

**Multiple episodes, currently in full remission**

**Continuous:** Symptoms fulfilling the diagnostic symptom criteria of the disorder are remaining for the majority of the illness course, with subthreshold symptom periods being very brief relative to the overall course.

**Unspecified**

*Specify* if:

**With catatonia** (refer to the criteria for catatonia associated with another mental disorder, [DSM-5] pp. 119–120, for definition).

**Coding note:** Use additional code 293.89 (F06.1) catatonia associated with schizophrenia to indicate the presence of the comorbid catatonia.

*Specify* current severity:

Severity is rated by a quantitative assessment of the primary symptoms of psychosis, including delusions, hallucinations, disorganized speech, abnormal psychomotor behavior, and negative symptoms. Each of these symptoms may be rated for its current severity (most severe in the last 7 days) on a 5-point scale ranging from 0 (not present) to 4 (present and severe). (See Clinician-Rated Dimensions of Psychosis Symptom Severity in the chapter "Assessment Measures" [in DSM-5].)

**Note:** Diagnosis of schizophrenia can be made without using this severity specifier.

## Criterion A

At least one of the two required symptoms must be delusions, hallucinations, or disorganized speech. These three are core "positive symptoms" that are diagnosed with high reliability and might reasonably be considered necessary for a diagnosis of schizophrenia. In DSM-IV, only one characteristic symptom was required if it was a bizarre delusion or "first-rank" hallucination. Because bizarre delusions and first-rank hallucinations have little diagnostic specificity and their reliability is poor (Bell et al. 2006), these "positive symptoms" are now treated like any other with regard to their diagnostic implication: as with other characteristic symptoms, two Criterion A symptoms need to be present for a diagnosis of schizophrenia. This change also eliminates the possibility that an individual with only catatonia and negative symptoms will receive a diagnosis of schizophrenia.

To better describe the nature of the affective abnormality in schizophrenia, the fifth characteristic type of symptoms in Criterion A—negative symptoms—has been changed from "affective flattening, alogia, or avolition" (as in DSM-IV) to "diminished emotional expression or avolition." This change to emphasize restricted affect should help clarify and more accurately describe the individual's presentation.

## Criterion B

Schizophrenia involves impairment in one or more major areas of functioning. Typically, functioning is clearly below prior levels of achievement, or, if the disturbance begins in childhood or adolescence, the expected level of functioning is not attained.

## Criterion C

Signs of the disturbance must persist continuously for at least 6 months. During at least 1 month of that time, symptoms must meet Criterion A (active-phase symptoms). Prodromal symptoms often proceed the active phase, and residual symptoms may follow. Some prodromal and residual symptoms are mild or subthreshold forms of hallucinations or delusions. Individuals may express a variety of unusual or odd beliefs that are not of delusional proportions; these are often referred to as "magical thinking" or "ideas of reference." The individual may report having unusual perceptual experiences, such as sensing the presence of an unseen person. The person's speech may be generally understandable but vague or digressive, while his or her behavior may be unusual but not grossly disorganized, such as muttering to oneself in public. Negative symptoms are common in the prodromal and residual phases and can be severe.

## Criterion D

Although mood symptoms and mood episodes are common and may be concurrent with active-phase symptoms, individuals with schizophrenia must have delusions or hallucinations in the absence of mood episodes, or the total duration of the mood episodes must be present for only a minority of the total duration of the active and residual periods of the illness. Otherwise, schizoaffective disorder may be the more appropriate diagnosis.

## Criterion E

Before making a diagnosis of schizophrenia, the clinician must rule out a wide variety of medical conditions that can present with psychotic symptoms, and must exclude drug-induced psychoses and psychoses attributable to delirium or other medical conditions (e.g., epilepsy, brain tumors, inflammatory brain disorders).

## Criterion F

If the individual has a history of autism spectrum disorder or a communication disorder of childhood onset, the additional diagnosis of schizophrenia is made only if prominent delusions or hallucinations, and the other required symptoms of schizophrenia, have been present for at least 1 month (or less if successfully treated).

## Specifiers

Multiple specifiers are provided to better describe the individual's course of illness. Catatonia may be specified if the full syndrome is present. Catatonic behaviors that may have previously led to the diagnosis of a catatonic subtype of schizophrenia are now covered in Criterion A4, which involves the presence of "grossly disorganized or catatonic behavior." The following additional diagnostic categories should be considered if the individual's symptoms are predominantly catatonic: catatonia associated with another mental disorder, catatonic disorder due to another medical condition, and unspecified catatonia.

# Schizoaffective Disorder

*Schizoaffective* is a term first used by Jacob Kasanin (1933) to describe a small group of severely ill patients with a mix of psychotic and mood symptoms. In DSM-5, the hallmark of schizoaffective disorder is the presence of either a major depressive or a manic mood episode concurrent with psychotic symptoms that meet schizophrenia Criterion A, such as hallucinations, delusions, disorganized speech, grossly disorganized or catatonic behavior, or negative symptoms. Additionally, mood symptoms must be a *prominent* feature of the condition and not a minor aspect. Other causes of these symptoms, including other medical conditions, substances of abuse, and medications, must be ruled out. The symptoms typically present together, or sometimes in an alternating fashion; psychotic symptoms may be mood-congruent or mood-incongruent.

Although schizoaffective disorder has long filled an important role in psychiatric practice, the diagnosis has suffered from low reliability. This situation began in 1980 when the diagnosis was included in DSM-III but had no operational criteria. Instead, two clinical vignettes were described in which the diagnosis was used. Criteria were introduced in DSM-III-R, and these continued mostly unchanged through DSM-IV. The criteria indicated that the mood symptoms had to be present for a "substantial portion of the total duration" of the illness; however, little guidance was given to help clinicians judge how long the duration of the mood symptoms should be relative to the duration of the illness. This gap has now been addressed: a major mood episode must be present for the majority of the total duration of the active and residual portions of the illness (i.e., the time since Criterion A has been met). This change should help clarify the boundaries of the disorder by providing guidance to the clinician about the proportion of time the patient experiences a mood syndrome.

---

## Diagnostic Criteria for Schizoaffective Disorder

---

A. An uninterrupted period of illness during which there is a major mood episode (major depressive or manic) concurrent with Criterion A of schizophrenia.
   **Note:** The major depressive episode must include Criterion A1: Depressed mood.
B. Delusions or hallucinations for 2 or more weeks in the absence of a major mood episode (depressive or manic) during the lifetime duration of the illness.
C. Symptoms that meet criteria for a major mood episode are present for the majority of the total duration of the active and residual portions of the illness.
D. The disturbance is not attributable to the effects of a substance (e.g., a drug of abuse, a medication) or another medical condition.

*Specify* whether:
   **295.70 (F25.0) Bipolar type:** This subtype applies if a manic episode is part of the presentation. Major depressive episodes may also occur.
   **295.70 (F25.1) Depressive type:** This subtype applies if only major depressive episodes are part of the presentation.

*Specify* if:
   **With catatonia** (refer to the criteria for catatonia associated with another mental disorder, [DSM-5] pp. 119–120, for definition).
      **Coding note:** Use additional code 293.89 (F06.1) catatonia associated with schizoaffective disorder to indicate the presence of the comorbid catatonia.

*Specify* if:
The following course specifiers are only to be used after a 1-year duration of the disorder and if they are not in contradiction to the diagnostic course criteria.
   **First episode, currently in acute episode:** First manifestation of the disorder meeting the defining diagnostic symptom and time criteria. An *acute episode* is a time period in which the symptom criteria are fulfilled.
   **First episode, currently in partial remission:** *Partial remission* is a time period during which an improvement after a previous episode is maintained and in which the defining criteria of the disorder are only partially fulfilled.
   **First episode, currently in full remission:** *Full remission* is a period of time after a previous episode during which no disorder-specific symptoms are present.
   **Multiple episodes, currently in acute episode:** Multiple episodes may be determined after a minimum of two episodes (i.e., after a first episode, a remission and a minimum of one relapse).
   **Multiple episodes, currently in partial remission**
   **Multiple episodes, currently in full remission**
   **Continuous:** Symptoms fulfilling the diagnostic symptom criteria of the disorder are remaining for the majority of the illness course, with subthreshold symptom periods being very brief relative to the overall course.
   **Unspecified**

*Specify* current severity:

Severity is rated by a quantitative assessment of the primary symptoms of psychosis, including delusions, hallucinations, disorganized speech, abnormal psychomotor behavior, and negative symptoms. Each of these symptoms may be rated for its current severity (most severe in the last 7 days) on a 5-point scale ranging from 0 (not present) to 4 (present and severe). (See Clinician-Rated Dimensions of Psychosis Symptom Severity in the chapter "Assessment Measures" [in DSM-5].)

**Note:** Diagnosis of schizoaffective disorder can be made without using this severity specifier.

## Criterion A

The presence of psychotic and mood symptoms is the essence of schizoaffective disorder. There must be an uninterrupted period in which major depressive or manic symptoms must be concurrent with Criterion A (of schizophrenia) psychotic symptoms. In fact, for many if not most individuals, the actual duration of the symptom overlap is a matter of months or years, not days or weeks.

## Criterion B

An important change in DSM-5 is that psychotic symptoms have to be present for 2 or more weeks in the absence of a major mood episode (depressive or manic) "during the lifetime duration of the illness" rather than "during the same period of illness" as in DSM IV. This change was prompted by the goal of making explicit that the diagnosis of schizoaffective disorder is based on the assessment of psychotic and mood symptoms during the lifetime duration of the illness. DSM-IV implied that a "period of illness" could refer, at a minimum, to a single *episode* of illness lasting at least 1 month (to meet Criterion A) or, at a maximum, to the *lifetime duration* of the illness. To increase reliability, the authors of DSM-IV restricted the diagnosis to a given episode. This resulted in a person's receiving a diagnosis of schizoaffective disorder, schizophreniform disorder, schizophrenia, or even a psychotic mood disorder at various times during the illness.

## Criterion C

The DSM-IV phrase "substantial portion of the total duration of the active and residual periods of the illness" has been replaced with "majority of the total duration of the active and residual portions, of the illness." The change was necessary because of the low reliability of the criterion and its limited clinical utility. Furthermore, the relative proportion of mood and psychotic symptoms can change over time, and clinicians and researchers often used different thresholds when applying this criterion. Researchers in several large studies had set the figure at 30% for total duration of their mood episodes (relative to the total duration of psychosis), but after examining field trial data the Psychotic Disorders Work Group recommended a threshold set at ≥50% as indicated by the word *majority.* Also new to DSM-5, Criterion C requires the assessment of mood symptoms not only during a current period of illness but over the entire course of a psychotic illness. If the mood symptoms are present for only a relatively brief period of time, the diagnosis is schizophrenia rather than schizoaffective disorder. When deciding whether an individual meets Criterion C, the clinician should review the total duration of psychotic illness (i.e., both active and residual symptoms) and determine when significant mood symptoms (untreated or in need of treatment with antidepressant and/or mood-stabilizing medication) accompanied the psychotic symptoms. This requires historical information and clinical judgment. For example, an individual with a 4-year history of active and residual symptoms of schizophrenia develops depressive and manic episodes that, taken together, do not occupy more than 1 year during the 4-year history of psychotic illness. This presentation would not meet Criterion C. The diagnosis in this example is schizophrenia, with the additional diagnosis of major depressive disorder to indicate the superimposed depressive episode.

### Criterion D

Medical illnesses, medications, and drugs of abuse need to be ruled out as a cause of the disturbance.

### Subtypes and Specifiers

The clinician may indicate whether the presentation includes a manic episode (bipolar type) or whether only major depressive episodes occur (depressive type). The presence of catatonia may be specified, as may course and current severity.

# Substance/Medication-Induced Psychotic Disorder

The essential feature of substance/medication-induced psychotic disorder is that the delusions or hallucinations (Criterion A) are judged to be causally related to the effects of a substance or medication because they have developed during or soon after substance intoxication or withdrawal, or following exposure to a medication (Criterion B). Last, the disturbance is not better explained by an independent psychotic disorder (Criterion C). The criteria have been edited for clarity and readability but are otherwise unchanged from DSM-IV. The diagnosis is used when the symptoms are in *excess* of those associated with an intoxication or withdrawal syndrome. For example, because hallucinations can occur during an alcohol withdrawal delirium, an additional diagnosis of a substance-induced psychotic disorder is not appropriate.

The diagnosis is common among persons who abuse substances, as well as in hospitals and clinics, where medications are often the cause of induced psychotic symptoms. The initiation of the disorder varies considerably depending on the substance and its pharmacological properties. For example, smoking a high dose of cocaine may produce psychosis within minutes, but days or weeks of high doses of alcohol or sedatives may be required to produce psychosis. Hallucinations may occur in any modality, but in the absence of a delirium they are often auditory. Alcohol-induced psychotic disorder usually occurs only after heavy prolonged use (generally years) in individuals with an alcohol use disorder. Stimulant medications are known to produce persecutory delusions, which may develop rapidly following the use of the stimulant (e.g., amphetamine, methamphetamine). Induced psychotic disorders usually resolve when the offending agent is withdrawn, although in some cases they can persist for weeks or months even when the person is treated with antipsychotic medications.

The diagnostic code recorded depends on the class of the substance. Further specifications include whether the symptoms had an onset during intoxication or withdrawal, and current severity.

## Diagnostic Criteria for Substance/Medication-Induced Psychotic Disorder

A. Presence of one or both of the following symptoms:

1. Delusions.
2. Hallucinations.

B. There is evidence from the history, physical examination, or laboratory findings of both (1) and (2):

1. The symptoms in Criterion A developed during or soon after substance intoxication or withdrawal or after exposure to a medication.
2. The involved substance/medication is capable of producing the symptoms in Criterion A.

C. The disturbance is not better explained by a psychotic disorder that is not substance/medication-induced. Such evidence of an independent psychotic disorder could include the following:

The symptoms preceded the onset of the substance/medication use; the symptoms persist for a substantial period of time (e.g., about 1 month) after the cessation of acute withdrawal or severe intoxication; or there is other evidence of an independent non-substance/medication-induced psychotic disorder (e.g., a history of recurrent non-substance/medication-related episodes).

D. The disturbance does not occur exclusively during the course of a delirium.

E. The disturbance causes clinically significant distress or impairment in social, occupational, or other important areas of functioning.

**Note:** This diagnosis should be made instead of a diagnosis of substance intoxication or substance withdrawal only when the symptoms in Criterion A predominate in the clinical picture and when they are sufficiently severe to warrant clinical attention.

**Coding note:** The ICD-9-CM and ICD-10-CM codes for the [specific substance/medication]-induced psychotic disorders are indicated in the table below. Note that the ICD-10-CM code depends on whether or not there is a comorbid substance use disorder present for the same class of substance. If a mild substance use disorder is comorbid with the substance-induced psychotic disorder, the 4th position character is "1," and the clinician should record "mild [substance] use disorder" before the substance-induced psychotic disorder (e.g., "mild cocaine use disorder with cocaine-induced psychotic disorder"). If a moderate or severe substance use disorder is comorbid with the substance-induced psychotic disorder, the 4th position character is "2," and the clinician should record "moderate [substance] use disorder" or "severe [substance] use disorder," depending on the severity of the comorbid substance use disorder. If there is no comorbid substance use disorder (e.g., after a one-time heavy use of the substance), then the 4th position character is "9," and the clinician should record only the substance-induced psychotic disorder.

| | ICD-9-CM | ICD-10-CM | | |
|---|---|---|---|---|
| | | With use disorder, mild | With use disorder, moderate or severe | Without use disorder |
| Alcohol | 291.9 | F10.159 | F10.259 | F10.959 |
| Cannabis | 292.9 | F12.159 | F12.259 | F12.959 |
| Phencyclidine | 292.9 | F16.159 | F16.259 | F16.959 |
| Other hallucinogen | 292.9 | F16.159 | F16.259 | F16.959 |
| Inhalant | 292.9 | F18.159 | F18.259 | F18.959 |
| Sedative, hypnotic, or anxiolytic | 292.9 | F13.159 | F13.259 | F13.959 |
| Amphetamine (or other stimulant) | 292.9 | F15.159 | F15.259 | F15.959 |
| Cocaine | 292.9 | F14.159 | F14.259 | F14.959 |
| Other (or unknown) substance | 292.9 | F19.159 | F19.259 | F19.959 |

*Specify* if (see Table 1 in the chapter "Substance-Related and Addictive Disorders" [in DSM-5] for diagnoses associated with substance class):
   **With onset during intoxication:** If the criteria are met for intoxication with the substance and the symptoms develop during intoxication.
   **With onset during withdrawal:** If the criteria are met for withdrawal from the substance and the symptoms develop during, or shortly after, withdrawal.
*Specify* current severity:
   Severity is rated by a quantitative assessment of the primary symptoms of psychosis, including delusions, hallucinations, abnormal psychomotor behavior, and negative symptoms. Each of these symptoms may be rated for its current severity (most severe in the last 7 days) on a 5-point scale ranging from 0 (not present) to 4 (present and severe). (See Clinician-Rated Dimensions of Psychosis Symptom Severity in the chapter "Assessment Measures" [in DSM-5].)
   **Note:** Diagnosis of substance/medication-induced psychotic disorder can be made without using this severity specifier.

# Criterion A

In DSM-IV, if a person realized that his or her hallucinations were substance or medication induced, the hallucinations were not counted toward this diagnosis, but this no longer applies.

## Criterion B

The delusions and/or hallucinations must have developed "during or soon after" substance intoxication or withdrawal or after other exposure to a medication, and the substance/medication involved must be "capable" of producing the psychosis. This language is more specific than in DSM-IV, which used the phrase "etiologically related."

## Criteria C, D, and E

This criterion outlines situations that cast doubt on a putative relationship between the use of a substance and the psychosis. For example, if the symptoms were present before the onset of substance or medication use, it is likely the psychosis is not substance induced. Delirium has been excluded as a cause of the psychosis, in which case the delirium would be separately coded. The disturbance must cause clinically significant distress or impairment.

# Psychotic Disorder Due to Another Medical Condition

This diagnosis is relatively unchanged from DSM-IV except for the addition of Criterion E to acknowledge the presence of significant distress or impairment. In addition, there must be evidence that the disorder is the direct pathophysiological consequence of another medical condition, and the disorder must not occur exclusively in the course of a delirium (otherwise the diagnosis is delirium). The code used is based on whether delusions or hallucinations are the predominant symptom. Further, the name of the medical disorder is included in the name of the mental disorder (e.g., psychotic disorder due to malignant lung neoplasm). Current severity can also be recorded.

Diagnostic Criteria for Psychotic Disorder Due to
Another Medical Condition

A. Prominent hallucinations or delusions.
B. There is evidence from the history, physical examination, or laboratory findings that the disturbance is the direct pathophysiological consequence of another medical condition.
C. The disturbance is not better explained by another mental disorder.
D. The disturbance does not occur exclusively during the course of a delirium.
E. The disturbance causes clinically significant distress or impairment in social, occupational, or other important areas of functioning.
*Specify* whether:
Code based on predominant symptom:
　　**293.81 (F06.2) With delusions:** If delusions are the predominant symptom.
　　**293.82 (F06.0) With hallucinations:** If hallucinations are the predominant symptom.

**Coding note:** Include the name of the other medical condition in the name of the mental disorder (e.g., 293.81 [F06.2] psychotic disorder due to malignant lung neoplasm, with delusions). The other medical condition should be coded and listed separately immediately before the psychotic disorder due to the medical condition (e.g., 162.9 [C34.90] malignant lung neoplasm; 293.81 [F06.2] psychotic disorder due to malignant lung neoplasm, with delusions).

*Specify* current severity:

Severity is rated by a quantitative assessment of the primary symptoms of psychosis, including delusions, hallucinations, abnormal psychomotor behavior, and negative symptoms. Each of these symptoms may be rated for its current severity (most severe in the last 7 days) on a 5-point scale ranging from 0 (not present) to 4 (present and severe). (See Clinician-Rated Dimensions of Psychosis Symptom Severity in the chapter "Assessment Measures" [in DSM-5].)

**Note:** Diagnosis of psychotic disorder due to another medical condition can be made without using this severity specifier.

# Catatonia Associated With Another Mental Disorder (Catatonia Specifier)

Catatonia associated with another mental disorder (catatonia specifier) may be used when criteria are met for catatonia during the course of a neurodevelopmental, psychotic, bipolar, depressive, or other mental disorder. The catatonia specifier is appropriate when the clinical picture is characterized by marked psychomotor disturbance and involves at least 3 of the 12 diagnostic features listed in Criterion A.

While catatonia occurs in over one-third of schizophrenia cases, the majority of catatonia cases occur in patients with a mood disorder. For this reason, catatonia was added as an episode specifier for the major mood disorders in DSM-IV. Catatonic symptoms need to be recognized because they have prognostic and treatment implications. The presence of neuroleptic malignant syndrome should be ruled out because of the serious nature of its complications.

The name of the associated mental disorder should be included when recording the name of the disorder (e.g., catatonia associated with schizoaffective disorder).

## Diagnostic Criteria for Catatonia Associated With Another Mental Disorder (Catatonia Specifier)          **293.89 (F06.1)**

A. The clinical picture is dominated by three (or more) of the following symptoms:

   1. Stupor (i.e., no psychomotor activity; not actively relating to environment).
   2. Catalepsy (i.e., passive induction of a posture held against gravity).
   3. Waxy flexibility (i.e., slight, even resistance to positioning by examiner).
   4. Mutism (i.e., no, or very little, verbal response [exclude if known aphasia]).
   5. Negativism (i.e., opposition or no response to instructions or external stimuli).
   6. Posturing (i.e., spontaneous and active maintenance of a posture against gravity).

7. Mannerism (i.e., odd, circumstantial caricature of normal actions).
8. Stereotypy (i.e., repetitive, abnormally frequent, non-goal-directed movements).
9. Agitation, not influenced by external stimuli.
10. Grimacing.
11. Echolalia (i.e., mimicking another's speech).
12. Echopraxia (i.e., mimicking another's movements).

**Coding note:** Indicate the name of the associated mental disorder when recording the name of the condition (i.e., 293.89 [F06.1] catatonia associated with major depressive disorder). Code first the associated mental disorder (e.g., neurodevelopmental disorder, brief psychotic disorder, schizophreniform disorder, schizophrenia, schizoaffective disorder, bipolar disorder, major depressive disorder, or other mental disorder) (e.g., 295.70 [F25.1] schizoaffective disorder, depressive type; 293.89 [F06.1] catatonia associated with schizoaffective disorder).

# Catatonic Disorder Due to Another Medical Condition

Catatonic disorder due to another medical condition has been moved from the DSM-IV chapter "Mental Disorders Due to a General Medical Condition." Catatonia has generally been viewed as a subtype of schizophrenia, as reflected in DSM-IV, but research has shown that catatonic symptoms can result from several medical disorders. For that reason, catatonic disorder due to a general medical condition was added as a new category in DSM-IV. The criteria for this disorder have changed to reflect greater specificity in the symptoms and impairment caused by the condition.

## Diagnostic Criteria for Catatonic Disorder Due to Another Medical Condition                               **293.89 (F06.1)**

A. The clinical picture is dominated by three (or more) of the following symptoms:

1. Stupor (i.e., no psychomotor activity; not actively relating to environment).
2. Catalepsy (i.e., passive induction of a posture held against gravity).
3. Waxy flexibility (i.e., slight, even resistance to positioning by examiner).
4. Mutism (i.e., no, or very little, verbal response [**Note:** not applicable if there is an established aphasia]).
5. Negativism (i.e., opposition or no response to instructions or external stimuli).
6. Posturing (i.e., spontaneous and active maintenance of a posture against gravity).
7. Mannerism (i.e., odd, circumstantial caricature of normal actions).
8. Stereotypy (i.e., repetitive, abnormally frequent, non-goal-directed movements).
9. Agitation, not influenced by external stimuli.
10. Grimacing.
11. Echolalia (i.e., mimicking another's speech).
12. Echopraxia (i.e., mimicking another's movements).

B. There is evidence from the history, physical examination, or laboratory findings that the disturbance is the direct pathophysiological consequence of another medical condition.

C. The disturbance is not better explained by another mental disorder (e.g., a manic episode).

D. The disturbance does not occur exclusively during the course of a delirium.

E. The disturbance causes clinically significant distress or impairment in social, occupational, or other important areas of functioning.

**Coding note:** Include the name of the medical condition in the name of the mental disorder (e.g., 293.89 [F06.1]) catatonic disorder due to hepatic encephalopathy). The other medical condition should be coded and listed separately immediately before the catatonic disorder due to the medical condition (e.g., 572.2 [K71.90] hepatic encephalopathy; 293.89 [F06.1] catatonic disorder due to hepatic encephalopathy).

## Criterion A

This criterion requires the presence of 3 or more of 12 symptoms typical for catatonia. In DSM-IV, the criteria were unclear as to how many symptoms were required.

## Criteria B and C

Because catatonic symptoms have been associated with a variety of medical disorders, medical conditions apart from the disorder in question need to be ruled out as a cause. This entails a detailed medical workup to rule out neurological, infectious, and other potential causes of the symptoms. For example, before concluding that the catatonia resulted from a herpes-related encephalopathy, the clinician should rule out brain tumors and other mass lesions.

Catatonic symptoms can occur in the context of other major mental disorders, such as mania, and these disorders need to be ruled out as well.

## Criteria D and E

If the symptoms occur only in the context of a delirium, then delirium is the appropriate diagnosis. This criterion is new to DSM-5 and specifies that the symptoms cause significant distress or impairment in social, occupational, and other important areas of functioning.

# Unspecified Catatonia

Catatonic syndromes can occur within the context of many other disorders, including psychotic disorders, depressive and bipolar disorders, and general medical conditions. In DSM-5, catatonia is no longer listed as a specific subtype of schizophrenia, but the text recognizes catatonic disorder as being due to another medical condition, as a specifier for a psychotic disorder or a depressive or bipolar disorder, or as an unspecified catatonia.

## Unspecified Catatonia

This category applies to presentations in which symptoms characteristic of catatonia cause clinically significant distress or impairment in social, occupational, or other important areas of functioning but either the nature of the underlying mental disorder or other medical condition is unclear, full criteria for catatonia are not met, or there is insufficient information to make a more specific diagnosis (e.g., in emergency room settings).

**Coding note:** Code first **781.99 (R29.818)** other symptoms involving nervous and musculoskeletal systems, followed by **293.89 (F06.1)** unspecified catatonia.

The diagnosis unspecified catatonia may be used when individuals with catatonic symptoms have clinically significant distress or impairment but the nature of the underlying mental disorder or other medical condition is unclear, the full criteria for catatonic disorder are not met, or there is insufficient information to make a more specific diagnosis.

# Other Specified Schizophrenia Spectrum and Other Psychotic Disorder and Unspecified Schizophrenia Spectrum and Other Psychotic Disorder

Other specified and unspecified schizophrenia spectrum and other psychotic disorders are residual categories for individuals whose symptoms do not fit within one of the more specific categories. The categories replace DSM-IV's psychotic disorder not otherwise specified.

Other specified schizophrenia spectrum and other psychotic disorder can be used in situations in which an individual has symptoms characteristic of a spectrum disorder that cause distress or impairment but that do not meet full criteria for a more specific disorder. In this case, the clinician chooses to communicate the reason that individual's symptoms do not meet the criteria. Specific examples are given in DSM-5 to describe situations in which this diagnosis may be appropriate. The category unspecified schizophrenia spectrum and other psychotic disorder is used when the clinician chooses not to specify the reason that criteria are not met for a more specific disorder, or when there is insufficient information to make a more specific diagnosis.

## Other Specified Schizophrenia Spectrum and Other Psychotic Disorder       **298.8** (F28)

This category applies to presentations in which symptoms characteristic of a schizophrenia spectrum and other psychotic disorder that cause clinically significant distress or impairment in social, occupational, or other important areas of functioning predominate but do not meet the full criteria for any of the disorders in the schizophrenia spectrum and other psychotic disorders diagnostic class. The other specified schizophrenia spectrum and other psychotic disorder category is used in situations in which the clinician chooses to communicate the specific reason that the presentation does not meet the criteria for any specific schizophrenia spectrum and other psychotic disorder. This is done by recording "other specified schizophrenia spectrum and other psychotic disorder" followed by the specific reason (e.g., "persistent auditory hallucinations").

Examples of presentations that can be specified using the "other specified" designation include the following:

1. **Persistent auditory hallucinations** occurring in the absence of any other features.
2. **Delusions with significant overlapping mood episodes:** This includes persistent delusions with periods of overlapping mood episodes that are present for a substantial portion of the delusional disturbance (such that the criterion stipulating only brief mood disturbance in delusional disorder is not met).
3. **Attenuated psychosis syndrome:** This syndrome is characterized by psychotic-like symptoms that are below a threshold for full psychosis (e.g., the symptoms are less severe and more transient, and insight is relatively maintained).
4. **Delusional symptoms in partner of individual with delusional disorder:** In the context of a relationship, the delusional material from the dominant partner provides content for delusional belief by the individual who may not otherwise entirely meet criteria for delusional disorder.

---

## Unspecified Schizophrenia Spectrum and Other Psychotic Disorder                                      298.9 (F29)

This category applies to presentations in which symptoms characteristic of a schizophrenia spectrum and other psychotic disorder that cause clinically significant distress or impairment in social, occupational, or other important areas of functioning predominate but do not meet the full criteria for any of the disorders in the schizophrenia spectrum and other psychotic disorders diagnostic class. The unspecified schizophrenia spectrum and other psychotic disorder category is used in situations in which the clinician chooses *not* to specify the reason that the criteria are not met for a specific schizophrenia spectrum and other psychotic disorder, and includes presentations in which there is insufficient information to make a more specific diagnosis (e.g., in emergency room settings).

# Clinician-Rated Dimensions of Psychosis Symptom Severity

The Clinician-Rated Dimensions of Psychosis Symptom Severity is available to help the clinician make detailed assessments of individuals across important domains, including hallucinations, delusions, disorganized speech, abnormal psychomotor behavior, negative symptoms, impaired cognition, depression, and mania. This instrument is described in the DSM-5 chapter "Assessment Measures."

# KEY POINTS

- Chapter organization has changed so that schizophrenia spectrum and other psychotic disorders are arranged along a gradient from least to most severe. Severity is defined by the level, number, and duration of psychotic signs and symptoms.

- Schizotypal personality disorder has been included in the schizophrenia spectrum, but the criteria and text remain in the personality disorders chapter. Evidence has accumulated since its initial description in DSM-III confirming its close etiological relationship with schizophrenia and other psychotic disorders.

- In the criteria for delusional disorder, the adjective *nonbizarre* has been removed (Criterion A), and the somatic subtype has been edited to ensure that individuals with a delusion regarding a physical defect are more appropriately diagnosed with body dysmorphic disorder.

- The diagnosis shared psychotic disorder has been eliminated because it was infrequently used and persons with the diagnosis generally had symptoms that met criteria for some other psychotic disorder (e.g., delusional disorder).

- With schizophrenia, bizarre delusions and "first-rank" hallucinations are no longer accorded special treatment. Further, clinicians will no longer record schizophrenia subtypes; despite historical precedent, there is scant research evidence supporting their clinical utility or predictive validity.

- The criteria for schizoaffective disorder now clarify that mood symptoms must constitute the "majority of the total duration of the active and residual portions of the illness." The change was necessary because of the low reliability and limited clinical utility of the wording in DSM-IV.

# References

American Psychiatric Association: Diagnostic and Statistical Manual of Mental Disorders, 4th Edition. Washington, DC, American Psychiatric Association, 1994

Bell V, Halligan PW, Ellis HD: Diagnosing delusions: a review of inter-rater reliability. Schizophr Res 86:76–79, 2006

Bleuler E: Dementia Praecox or the Group of Schizophrenias. Translated by Zinken J. New York, International Universities Press, 1950

Cermolacce M, Sass L, Parnas J: What is bizarre in bizarre delusions? A critical review. Schizophr Bull 36:667–679, 2010

Helmes E, Landmark J: Subtypes of schizophrenia: a cluster analytic approach. Can J Psychiatry 48:702–708, 2003

Kasanin J: The acute schizoaffective psychoses. Am J Psychiatry 90:97–126, 1933

Kraepelin E: Dementia Praecox and Paraphrenia. Translated by Barclay RM, Robertson GM. Edinburgh, E & S Livingstone, 1919

Langfeldt G: The Schizophreniform States: A Katamnestic Study Based on Individual Reexaminations. Copenhagen, Denmark, Munksgaard, 1939

McGlashan T, Fenton W: Classical Subtypes of Schizophrenia. Washington, DC, American Psychiatric Association, 1994

Nordgaard J, Arnfred SM, Handest P, et al: The diagnostic status of first-rank symptoms. Schizophr Bull 34:137–154, 2008

Schneider K: Clinical Psychopathology. New York, Grune & Stratton, 1959

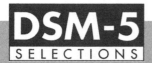

# Schizophrenia Spectrum and Other Psychotic Disorders

## DSM-5® Clinical Cases

# Introduction

*John W. Barnhill, M.D.*

Schizophrenia is the prototypical psychotic disorder. Not only is it the most common psychosis, but schizophrenia tends to involve abnormalities in all five of the emphasized symptom domains: hallucinations, delusions, disorganized thinking (speech), grossly disorganized or abnormal motor behavior (including catatonia), and negative symptoms. Like the DSM-5 neurodevelopmental disorders, schizophrenia is viewed as a neuropsychiatric disorder with complex genetics and a clinical course that tends to begin during a predictable stage of development. Whereas the neurodevelopmental disorders tend to begin during childhood, symptoms of schizophrenia tend to reliably develop during late adolescence and early adulthood.

The schizophrenia diagnosis has undergone some minor revisions for DSM-5. First, because of their limited diagnostic stability, low reliability, and poor validity, schizophrenia subtypes have been eliminated. They had included such categories as disorganized, paranoid, and residual types of schizophrenia.

Long associated with schizophrenia, catatonia remains one of the potential diagnostic criteria for most of the psychotic diagnoses, including schizophrenia, but it can now be designated as a specifier for other psychiatric and nonpsychiatric medical conditions, including depressive and bipolar disorders. "Other specified catatonia" can also be diagnosed when criteria are either uncertain or incomplete for either the catatonia or the comorbid psychiatric or nonpsychiatric medical condition.

The DSM-5 schizophrenia diagnosis requires persistence of two of five symptomatic criteria (delusions, hallucinations, disorganized speech, disorganized behavior or catatonia, and negative symptoms). One pertinent change is the elimination of a special status for particular types of delusions and hallucinations, any one of which would previously have been adequate to fulfill symptomatic criteria for schizophrenia. A second change is the requirement for one of the two symptomatic criteria to be a positive symptom, such as delusions, hallucinations, or disorganized thinking.

Criteria for schizoaffective disorder have been significantly tightened. As was the case in DSM-IV, a diagnosis of schizoaffective disorder requires that the patient meet criteria for schizophrenia and have symptoms of either major depressive or bipolar disorder concurrent with having active symptoms of schizophrenia. Also, as was the case previously, there must have been a 2-week period of delusions or hallucinations without prominent mood symptoms. The significant change is that in DSM-5 symptoms that meet criteria for a major mood disorder must be present for the majority of the total duration of the active and residual phases of the overall illness. Therefore, the DSM-5 schizoaffective diagnosis requires more attention to the longitudinal course than was previously the case. Furthermore, the diagnostic requirement that major mood symptoms be present during most of the course of the psychotic disorder (including both the acute and the residual phases) will likely lead to a significant reduction in the number of people who meet criteria for schizoaffective disorder.

Delusional disorder remains focused on the presence of delusions in the absence of other active symptoms of schizophrenia, depressive or bipolar disorders, and pertinent substance use. Bizarre delusions are now included as symptomatic criteria for delusional disorder, whereas delusions that are considered to be part of body dysmorphic disorder and obsessive-compulsive disorder should not lead to a delusional disorder diagnosis but rather to a primary diagnosis of either body dysmorphic disorder or obsessive-compulsive disorder, along with the "absent insight/delusional beliefs" specifier.

Brief psychotic disorder and schizophreniform disorder remain essentially unchanged in DSM-5. They remain distinguished from schizophrenia primarily on the basis of the duration of symptoms.

Not specifically discussed in this text are diagnoses that involve atypical or incomplete presentations or involve situations such as the emergency room setting where information is often incomplete. These include "other specified schizophrenia spectrum and other psychotic disorder," "unspecified catatonia," and "unspecified schizophrenia spectrum and other psychotic disorder."

These "other" diagnoses reflect the reality that humans' thoughts, feelings, and behaviors lie on a continuum, as do their disorders, and the "other" option is a diagnostic option through much of DSM-5. This diagnostic gray zone is particularly poignant in regard to schizophrenia spectrum illness. For many people who end up with a chronic illness such as schizophrenia or schizoaffective disorder, there exists a period of time in which they begin to show symptoms but are not yet diagnosed. It had been proposed that this issue be addressed in DSM-5 by creating a new diagnosis, *attenuated psychosis syndrome*. Psychiatrists are not yet able to robustly predict which patients are most likely to go on to develop full-blown psychotic symptoms, but accurate prediction is important enough that the syndrome is mentioned in two places in DSM-5. First, attenuated psychosis syndrome can be used as a specifier within this chapter of DSM-5, where it would be listed as "other specified schizophrenia spectrum and other disorders (attenuated psychosis syndrome)." The condition is also discussed in more detail among the "Conditions for Further Study."

## Suggested Readings

Bromet EJ, Kotov R, Fochtmann LJ, et al: Diagnostic shifts during the decade following first admission for psychosis. Am J Psychiatry 168(11):1186–1194, 2011

Lieberman JA, Murray RM: Comprehensive Care of Schizophrenia: A Textbook of Clinical Management, 2nd Edition. New York, Oxford University Press, 2012

Tamminga CA, Sirovatka PJ, Regier DA, et al (eds): Deconstructing Psychosis: Refining the Research Agenda for DSM-V. Arlington, VA, American Psychiatric Association, 2010

# Case 1: Emotionally Disturbed

*Carol A. Tamminga, M.D.*

Felicia Allen was a 32-year-old woman brought to the emergency room (ER) by police after she apparently tried to steal a bus. Because she appeared to be an "emotionally disturbed person," a psychiatry consultation was requested.

According to the police report, Ms. Allen threatened the driver with a knife, took control of the almost empty city bus, and crashed it. A more complete story was elicited from a friend of Ms. Allen's who had been on the bus but who had not been arrested. According to her, they had boarded the bus on their way to a nearby shopping mall. Ms. Allen became frustrated when the driver refused her dollar bills. She looked in her purse, but instead of finding exact change, she pulled out a kitchen knife that she carried for protection. The driver fled, so she got into the empty seat and drove the bus across the street into a nearby parked car.

On examination, Ms. Allen was a handcuffed, heavyset young woman with a bandage on her forehead. She fidgeted and rocked back and forth in her chair. She appeared to be mumbling to herself. When asked what she was saying, the patient made momentary eye contact and just repeated, "Sorry, sorry." She did not respond to other questions.

More information was elicited from a psychiatrist who had come to the ER soon after the accident. He said that Ms. Allen and her friend were longtime residents at the state psychiatric hospital where he worked. They had just begun to take passes every week as part of an effort toward social remediation; it had been Ms. Allen's first bus ride without a staff member.

According to the psychiatrist, Ms. Allen had received a diagnosis of "childhood-onset, treatment-resistant paranoid schizophrenia." She had started hearing voices by age 5 years. Big, strong, intrusive, and psychotic, she had been hospitalized almost constantly since age 11. Her auditory hallucinations generally consisted of a critical voice commenting on her behavior. Her thinking was concrete, but when relaxed she could be self-reflective. She was motivated to please and recurrently said her biggest goal was to "have my own room in my own house with my own friends." The psychiatrist said that he was not sure what had caused her to pull out the knife. She had not been hallucinating lately and had been feeling less paranoid, but he wondered if she had been more psychotic than she had let on. It was possible that she was just impatient and irritated. The psychiatrist also believed that she had spent almost no period of life developing normally and so had very little experience with the real world.

Ms. Allen had been taking clozapine for 1 year, with good resolution of her auditory hallucinations. She had gained 35 pounds during that time, but she had less trouble getting out of bed in the morning, was hoping that she could eventually get a job and live more independently, and had insisted on continuing to take the clozapine. The bus trip to the shopping mall was intended to be a step in that direction.

## Diagnosis

• Schizophrenia, multiple episodes, currently in active phase

## Discussion

Stealing a city bus is not reasonable, and it reflects Ms. Allen's inability to deal effectively with the world. Her thinking is concrete. She behaves bizarrely. She mumbles and talks to herself, suggesting auditory hallucinations. She lives in a state mental hospital, suggesting severe, persistent mental illness.

DSM-5 schizophrenia requires at least two of five symptoms: delusions, hallucinations, disorganized speech, disorganized or abnormal behavior, and negative symptoms. Functioning must be impaired, and continuous signs of the illness must persist for at least 6 months. Even without any more information about Ms. Allen's history, the diagnosis of schizophrenia is clear.

Ms. Allen's psychosis began when she was a child. Early-onset symptoms are often unrecognized because children tend to view their psychotic experience as "normal." Identifying the symptom (e.g., hearing voices that are not there) and associating this with a milestone (e.g., going to a certain grade or school) can help the adult patient retrospectively identify symptom onset. Although the symptoms and treatments are similar for both, childhood-onset schizophrenia is often more severe than adult-onset schizophrenia. Early psychotic symptoms are highly disruptive to normal childhood development. Florid psychotic symptoms are impairing in and of themselves, but they also deprive the young person of the social learning and cognitive development that take place during critical childhood years.

Ms. Allen's behavior on the bus likely reflects not only the psychosis and cognitive dysfunction that are part of schizophrenia but also her diminished experience in real-life social settings. In addition to treating her psychotic symptoms with clozapine, her psychiatric team appears to be trying to remediate her losses by connecting her to a "friend" and organizing the shopping trip. They are also quite active and involved, as reflected by the psychiatrist's almost immediate presence in the ER after the bus incident.

Schizophrenia is a heterogeneous disorder, affecting multiple domains. It is likely that there are multiple schizophrenias, differentiated by as yet unknown markers. Because of insufficient evidence about validity, DSM-5 has done away with categories such as schizophrenia, paranoid type. Instead, DSM-5 outlines several ways in which the diagnosis can be subtyped. One way is by overall activity and chronicity of symptoms (e.g., single vs. multiple episodes; in acute episode, in partial remission, in full remission). Another way to categorize is by assessing the severity of each of the five core schizophrenia symptoms, using a 0–4 scale.

For example, Ms. Allen was able to try to travel with a "friend," and her hospital-based psychiatrist did arrive in the ER very quickly. These might reflect an engaged, active treatment program, but when combined with her apologetic attitude and her stated efforts toward independence, they likely indicate a relative lack of negative symptoms such as anhedonia, reduced social networks, and alogia. Such activity-driven behavior is unusual in patients with schizophrenia and suggests that she is not depressed. It is hard to judge Ms. Allen's cognitive capacity without testing. Her obvious concrete thinking is represented by a failure to understand the process of paying for her bus ride or abstracting behavioral clues. Whether she has the additional characteristics of a schizophrenia-like working memory disorder or attentional dysfunction is hard to tell from this vignette, but she should be tested.

In addition to assessing the extent of positive symptoms, it is crucial for the field of psychiatry to better understand and categorize the negative symptoms and cognitive dysfunction of schizophrenia. Whereas the most effective interventions for schizophrenia have long revolved around the antipsychotic medications that ameliorate positive symptoms, future treatments will likely focus increasingly on the specific behavioral, cognitive, and emotional disturbances that are also an integral part of schizophrenia.

## Suggested Readings

Ahmed AO, Green BA, Goodrum NM, et al: Does a latent class underlie schizotypal personality disorder? Implications for schizophrenia. J Abnorm Psychol 122(2):475–491, 2013

Heckers S, Barch DM, Bustillo J, et al: Structure of the psychotic disorders classification in DSM 5. Schizophr Res 150(1):11–14, 2013

Tandon R, Gaebel W, Barch DM, et al: Definition and description of schizophrenia in the DSM-5. Schizophr Res 150(1):3–10, 2013

# Case 2: Increasingly Odd

*Ming T. Tsuang, M.D., Ph.D., D.Sc.*
*William S. Stone, Ph.D.*

Gregory Baker was a 20-year-old African American man who was brought to the emergency room (ER) by the campus police of the university from which he had been suspended several months earlier. The police had been called by a professor who reported that Mr. Baker had walked into his classroom shouting, "I am the Joker, and I am looking for Batman." When Mr. Baker refused to leave the class, the professor contacted security.

Although Mr. Baker had much academic success as a teenager, his behavior had become increasingly odd during the past year. He quit seeing his friends and spent most of his time lying in bed staring at the ceiling. He lived with several family members but rarely spoke to any of them. He had been suspended from college because of lack of attendance. His sister said that she had recurrently seen him mumbling quietly to himself and noted that he would sometimes, at night, stand on the roof of their home and wave his arms as if he were "conducting a symphony." He denied having any intention of jumping from the roof or having any thoughts of self-harm, but claimed that he felt liberated and in tune with the music when he was on the roof. Although his father and sister had tried to encourage him to see someone at the university's student health office, Mr. Baker had never seen a psychiatrist and had no prior hospitalizations.

During the prior several months, Mr. Baker had become increasingly preoccupied with a female friend, Anne, who lived down the street. While he insisted to his family that they were engaged, Anne told Mr. Baker's sister that they had hardly ever spoken and certainly were not dating. Mr. Baker's sister also reported that he had written many letters to Anne but never mailed them; instead, they just accumulated on his desk.

His family said that they had never known him to use illicit substances or alcohol, and his toxicology screen was negative. When asked about drug use, Mr. Baker appeared angry and did not answer.

On examination in the ER, Mr. Baker was a well-groomed young man who was generally uncooperative. He appeared constricted, guarded, inattentive, and preoccupied. He became enraged when the ER staff brought him dinner. He loudly insisted that all of the hospital's food was poisoned and that he would only drink a specific type of bottled water. He was noted to have paranoid, grandiose, and romantic delusions. He appeared to be internally preoccupied, although he denied hallucinations. Mr. Baker reported feeling "bad" but denied depression and had no disturbance in his sleep or appetite. He was oriented and spoke articulately but refused formal cognitive testing. His insight and judgment were deemed to be poor.

Mr. Baker's grandmother had died in a state psychiatric hospital, where she had lived for 30 years. Her diagnosis was unknown. Mr. Baker's mother was reportedly "crazy." She had abandoned the family when Mr. Baker was young, and he was raised by his father and paternal grandmother.

Ultimately, Mr. Baker agreed to sign himself into the psychiatric unit, stating, "I don't mind staying here. Anne will probably be there, so I can spend my time with her."

## Diagnosis

• Schizophrenia, first episode, currently in acute episode

## Discussion

Mr. Baker's case involves an all-too-familiar scenario in which a high-functioning young man undergoes a significant decline. In addition to having paranoid, grandiose, and romantic delusions, Mr. Baker appears to be responding to internal stimuli (i.e., auditory hallucinations) and demonstrating negative symptoms (lying in bed all day). These symptoms have persisted and intensified over the prior year. The history does not indicate medications, substances of abuse, or other medical or psychiatric disorders that could cause these symptoms. Therefore, he meets DSM-5 criteria for schizophrenia. Although a family history of psychiatric illness is not a requisite for his DSM-5 diagnosis, Mr. Baker's mother and grandmother appear to have also had major mental disorders.

Schizophrenia is, however, a heterogeneous disorder. For example, Mr. Baker's most prominent symptoms are delusions. Another person with schizophrenia might present most prominently with disorganization of speech and behavior and without any delusions. DSM-5 tries to address this heterogeneity by encouraging a dimensional viewpoint rather than a categorical one. In other words, instead of clarifying whether a patient has "paranoid" or "disorganized" schizophrenia, DSM-5 encourages an assessment of a variety of specifiers. One important specifier, the course specifier, requires a longitudinal assessment to determine whether this is a first episode or one of multiple episodes, and whether it is an acute episode, in partial remission, or in full remission.

DSM-5 also encourages specific ratings of symptoms. For example, is this schizophrenic episode accompanied by catatonia? On a 5-point scale (from 0 to 4), how severe is each of the five cardinal schizophrenia symptoms? DSM-5 also encourages an assessment of cognition, mania, and depression domains. For example, some of Mr. Baker's behaviors (e.g., interrupting a class to proclaim his identity as the Joker) may seem to be symptomatic of mania, but they are unaccompanied by disturbances in sleep, mood, or level of activity. Similarly, Mr. Baker said he felt "bad" but not depressed. These clinical observations likely distinguish Mr. Baker from other subcategories of people with schizophrenia.

The schizophrenia diagnosis can be made without assessing these severity specifiers. Nevertheless, the use of dimensional ratings improves the ability to assess Mr. Baker for the presence of core symptoms of schizophrenia in a more individualized manner. The inclusion of dimensions that cut across diagnostic categories will facilitate the development of a differential diagnosis that includes bipolar disorder and schizoaffective disorder. These assessments may clarify Mr. Baker's functional prognosis in major life roles (e.g., living arrangement or occupational status). Finally, repeated dimensional assessments may facilitate a longitudinal understanding of Mr. Baker's symptomatology, development, and likely responses to treatment.

## Suggested Readings

Barch DM, Bustillo J, Gaebel W, et al: Logic and justification for dimensional assessment of symptoms and related clinical phenomena in psychosis: relevance to DSM-5. Schizophr Res 150(1):15–20, 2013 PubMed ID: 23706415

Cuesta MJ, Basterra V, Sanchez-Torres A, et al: Controversies surrounding the diagnosis of schizophrenia and other psychoses. Expert Rev Neurother 9(10):1475–1486, 2009

Heckers S, Barch DM, Bustillo J, et al: Structure of the psychotic disorders classification in DSM 5. Schizophr Res 150(1):11–14, 2013

Tandon R, Gaebel W, Barch DM, et al: Definition and description of schizophrenia in the DSM-5. Schizophr Res 150(1):3–10, 2013

# Case 3: Hallucinations of a Spiritual Nature

*Lianne K. Morris Smith, M.D.*
*Dolores Malaspina, M.D., M.P.H.*

Hakim Coleman was a 25-year-old U.S. Army veteran turned community college student who presented to the emergency room (ER) with his girlfriend and sister. On examination, he was a tall, slim, and well-groomed young man with glasses. He spoke softly, with an increased latency of speech. His affect was blunted except when he became anxious while discussing his symptoms.

Mr. Coleman stated that he had come to the ER at his sister's suggestion. He said he could use a "general checkup" because of several days of "migraines" and "hallucinations of a spiritual nature" that had persisted for 3 months. His headache involved "sharp, shooting" sensations in various bilateral locations in his head and a "ringing" sensation along the midline of his brain that seemed to worsen when he thought about his vices.

Mr. Coleman described his vices as being "alcohol, cigarettes, disrespecting my parents, girls." He denied guilt, anxiety, or preoccupation about any of his military duties during his tour in Iraq, but he had joined an evangelical church 4 months earlier in the context of being "riddled with guilt" about "all the things I've done." Three months earlier, he began "hearing voices trying to make me feel guilty" most days. The last auditory hallucination had been the day before. During these past few months, he had noticed that strangers were commenting on his past sins.

Mr. Coleman believed that his migraines and guilt might be due to alcohol withdrawal. He had been drinking three or four cans of beer most days of the week for several years until he "quit" 4 months earlier after joining the church. He still drank "a beer or two" every other week but felt guilty afterward. He denied alcohol withdrawal symptoms such as tremor and sweats. He had smoked cannabis up to twice monthly for years but completely quit when he joined the church. He denied using other illicit drugs except for one uneventful use of cocaine 3 years earlier. He slept well except occasional nights when he would sleep only a few hours in order to finish an academic assignment.

Otherwise, Mr. Coleman denied depressive, manic, or psychotic symptoms and violent ideation. He denied posttraumatic stress disorder (PTSD) symptoms. Regarding stressors, he felt overwhelmed by his current responsibilities, which included attending school and near-daily church activities. He had been a straight-A student at the start of the school year but was now receiving Bs and Cs.

The patient's girlfriend and sister were interviewed separately. They agreed that Mr. Coleman had become socially isolative and quiet, after having previously been fun and outgoing. He had also never been especially religious prior to this episode. His sister believed that Mr. Coleman had been "brainwashed" by the church. His girlfriend, however, had attended services with Mr. Coleman. She reported that several members of the congregation had told her they had occasionally talked to new members who felt guilt over their prior behaviors, but none who had ever hallucinated, and they were worried about him.

A physical examination of the patient, including a neurological screen, was unremarkable, as were routine laboratory testing, a blood alcohol level, and urine toxicology. A noncontrast head computed tomography (CT) scan was normal.

## Diagnosis

• Schizophreniform disorder, provisional

## Discussion

The differential diagnosis for a young military veteran with new-onset psychosis and a history of substance abuse is broad. The primary possibilities include a primary psychotic disorder, a psychotic mood disorder, substance-induced psychosis, a psychotic disorder secondary to a general medical condition, a shared cultural syndrome, and PTSD.

Mr. Coleman seems most likely to fit a DSM-5 schizophreniform disorder, a diagnosis that differs from schizophrenia in two substantive ways: the total duration of schizophreniform illness—including prodrome, active, and residual phases—is greater than 1 month but less than 6 months. In addition, there is no criterion that mandates social or occupational impairment. For both schizophreniform disorder and schizophrenia, the patient must meet at least two of five symptomatic criteria. Mr. Coleman describes hallucinations ("hearing voices trying to make me feel guilty") and negative symptoms (blunted affect, avolition, social isolation). The case report does not mention delusions or disorganization of either speech or behavior.

Not relevant to DSM-5 criteria, but of interest, is that Mr. Coleman reports two schneiderian symptoms besides auditory hallucinations: ideas of reference and possible cenesthetic hallucinations based on his description of his atypical headaches ("ringing" in his brain).

DSM-5 indicates that depressive and manic symptoms should be explored as potentially causing the psychosis, and Mr. Coleman denies pertinent mood symptoms. The diagnosis of schizophreniform disorder also requires exclusion of a contributory general medical condition or substance use disorder. Mr. Coleman appears to have no medical complaints, and both his physical examination and laboratory testing are noncontributory.

The patient himself is convinced that his symptoms are due to alcohol. At its worst, however, his drinking appears to have been modest, and he has lately been drinking "a beer or two" every other week. He denies ever having had symptoms of withdrawal or other complications. His hallucinations began months after he cut back on his alcohol use, and they persisted for months. Additionally, his laboratory tests, including a hepatic panel and complete blood count, were normal, which would be unusual in patients with the sort of chronic alcohol use that usually accompanies alcohol-induced psychosis or significant withdrawal. Mr. Coleman's chronic cannabis use could potentially be implicated in the development of psychosis, but not only was his cannabis use sporadic, he apparently had not used for several months prior to the onset of hallucinations, and results of a toxicology screen were negative. It would appear that Mr. Coleman's concerns about alcohol and cannabis are linked to hyperreligious guilt rather than an actual substance use disorder. The possibility of a general medical condition was considered, but his normal laboratory testing and physical examination results provided no such evidence.

Schizophreniform disorders last at least 1 month but less than 6 months. In regard to Mr. Coleman, his initial 1–2 months of religious preoccupation and guilty ruminations would be considered a prodrome phase. The 3 months preceding presentation to the ER would represent the active phase of psychosis. Because Mr. Coleman's psychotic symptoms have lasted 4–5 months but are ongoing, he would be said to have provisional schizophreniform disorder. Obviously, everyone who goes on to develop schizophrenia has a 6-month period in which they could be said to have schizophreniform disorder, but about one-third of people with schizophreniform disorder do not go on to develop schizophrenia or schizoaffective disorder.

Three other diagnostic possibilities that deserve mention include PTSD, a dissociative disorder, and a shared cultural syndrome. The case does not go into depth about

Mr. Coleman's military experience, but simply the experience of being in an active war zone can be a traumatic exposure. He did not report features of PTSD, but it is not clear how extensively possible PTSD symptoms were discussed. Given that avoidance is a cardinal feature of PTSD—making it less likely that he would spontaneously report the symptoms without being prompted—it would be useful to tactfully explore the possibility.

Mr. Coleman's family members indicate that his symptoms began around the time of his initiation into an evangelical church and worry that he has been "brainwashed." DSM-5 includes a possibly pertinent category, listed under "other specified dissociative disorders," within the chapter on dissociative disorders. This disorder is reserved for individuals who experience an identity disturbance due to prolonged and coercive persuasion in the context of such experiences as long-term political imprisonment or recruitment by cults.

It is also possible that Mr. Coleman's unusual beliefs are a nonpathological manifestation of religious beliefs that he shares with other members of his church.

It appears that his psychotic symptoms began prior to his entry into the church, however, and may have been an underlying motivating factor for him to join a church that had previously not been of interest to him. In addition, although he attended church frequently, there is no evidence that he joined a cult or particularly manipulative religious sect. Furthermore, other congregants viewed his hallucinations as aberrant, indicating that his views were not part of a shared cultural or religious mindset.

The initial diagnosis of provisional schizophreniform disorder is temporary. Longitudinal follow-up will clarify whether Mr. Coleman's symptoms attenuate or progress to a chronic psychotic illness.

## Suggested Readings

Bromet EJ, Kotov R, Fochtmann LJ, et al: Diagnostic shifts during the decade following first admission for psychosis. Am J Psychiatry 168(11):1186–1194, 2011

Heckers S, Barch DM, Bustillo J, et al: Structure of the psychotic disorders classification in DSM 5. Schizophr Res 150(1):, 11–14, 2013

Tamminga CA, Sirovatka PJ, Regier DA, van Os J: Deconstructing Psychosis: Refining the Research Agenda for DSM-V. Arlington, VA, American Psychiatric Association, 2010

# Case 4: Mind Control

*Rajiv Tandon, M.D.*

Itsuki Daishi was a 23-year-old engineering student from Japan who was referred to his university student mental health clinic by a professor who had become concerned about his irregular school attendance. When they had met to discuss his declining performance, Mr. Daishi had volunteered to the professor that he was distracted by the "listening devices" and "thought control machines" that had been placed in his apartment.

While initially wary of talking to the psychiatrist, Mr. Daishi indicated that he was relieved to finally get a chance to talk in a room that had not yet been bugged. He said that his problems began 3 months earlier, after he returned from a visit to Japan. He said his first indication of trouble was that his classmates sneezed and grinned in an odd way when he entered the classroom. One day when returning from class, he noticed two strangers outside his apartment and wondered why they were there.

Mr. Daishi said that he first noticed that his apartment had been bugged about a week after the strangers had been standing outside his apartment. When he watched television, he noticed that reporters commented indirectly and critically about him. This experience was most pronounced when he watched Fox News, which he believed had targeted him because of his "superior intelligence" and his intention to someday become the prime minister of Japan. He believed that Fox News was trying to make him "go mad" by instilling conservative ideas into his brain, and that this was possible through the use of tiny mind-control devices they had installed in his apartment.

Mr. Daishi's sleep became increasingly irregular as he became more vigilant, and he feared that everyone at school and in his apartment complex was "in on the plot." He became withdrawn and stopped attending classes, but he continued to eat and maintain his personal hygiene.

He denied feeling elated or euphoric. He described his level of energy as "okay" and his thinking as clear "except when they try to put ideas into my head." He admitted to feeling extremely fearful for several hours on one occasion during his recent trip to Japan. At that time, he had smoked "a lot of pot" and began hearing strange sounds and believing that his friends were laughing at him. He denied any cannabis consumption since his return to the United States and denied ever having experimented with any other substances of abuse, saying that he generally would not even drink alcohol. He denied all other history of auditory or visual hallucinations.

When Mr. Daishi's uncle, listed as his local guardian, was contacted, he described his nephew as a healthy, intelligent, and somewhat shy boy without any prior history of any major psychiatric illness. He described Mr. Daishi's parents as very loving and supportive, although his father "might be a little stern." There was no family history of any major mental illness.

On examination, Mr. Daishi was well groomed and cooperative, with normal psychomotor activity. His speech was coherent and goal directed. He described his mood as "afraid." The range and mobility of his affective expression were normal. He denied any ideas of guilt, suicide, or worthlessness. He was convinced that he was being continuously monitored and that there were "mind-control" devices in his apartment. He denied hallucinations. His cognitive functions were grossly within normal limits. He appeared to have no insight into his beliefs.

On investigation, Mr. Daishi's laboratory test results were normal, his head computed tomography scan was unremarkable, and his urine drug screen was negative for any substances of abuse.

## Diagnosis

- Delusional disorder, mixed type

## Discussion

Mr. Daishi meets criteria for delusional disorder, which requires one or more delusions that persist for greater than 1 month but no other psychotic symptoms. Most of Mr. Daishi's delusions are persecutory and related to monitoring devices. He has delusions of reference (classmates sneezing and grinning at him), persecution ("trying to make me go mad," monitoring devices), and thought insertion ("machines trying to put ideas into my head"). He warrants the "mixed" specifier because the apparent motivation for his having been targeted appears to be grandiose (his "superior intelligence" and plans to be the prime minister of Japan), but he has no other symptoms of mania.

Other psychotic disorders should also be considered. The 3-month duration of symptoms is too long for brief psychotic disorder (no longer than 1 month) and too brief for schizophrenia (no briefer than 6 months) but is an appropriate duration for schizophreniform disorder (between 1 and 6 months' duration). Mr. Daishi does not appear, however, to have a second symptom (e.g., hallucinations, negative symptoms, or disorganization) as required for a schizophreniform diagnosis. In DSM-IV, a single bizarre delusion—the delusion of thought insertion—would have been adequate to reach symptomatic criteria for schizophreniform disorder (or schizophrenia), but bizarre delusions no longer receive special treatment among the DSM-5 schizophrenia spectrum disorders.

The absence of manic or major depressive mood symptoms excludes a diagnosis of bipolar disorder (with psychotic symptoms), major depressive disorder (with psychotic symptoms), or schizoaffective disorder.

Substance-induced psychotic disorder should be considered in view of Mr. Daishi's recent, significant cannabis consumption. His symptoms do seem to have developed soon after consumption of a substance known to cause psychosis (cannabis, with or without adulteration with another substance such as phencyclidine), and cannabis might be considered a trigger that Mr. Daishi should avoid in the future. DSM-5 specifically excludes the diagnosis of substance-induced psychotic disorder, however, when symptoms persist for a substantial period of time (e.g., 1 month) following the discontinuation of the substance.

## Suggested Readings

Cermolacce M, Sass L, Parnas J: What is bizarre about bizarre delusions? A critical review. Schizophr Bull 36(4):667–679, 2010

Nordgaard J, Arnfred SM, Handest P, et al: The diagnostic status of first-rank symptoms. Schizophr Bull 34(1):137–154, 2008

Tandon R: The nosology of schizophrenia: toward DSM-5 and ICD-11. Psychiatr Clin North Am 35(3):557–569, 2012

Tandon R, Carpenter WT: DSM-5 status of psychotic disorders: 1 year prepublication. Schizophr Bull 38(3):369–370, 2012

# Case 5: Sad and Psychotic

*Stephan Heckers, M.D., M.Sc.*

John Evans was a 25-year-old single, unemployed white man who had been see-ing a psychiatrist for several years for management of psychosis, depression, anxiety, and abuse of marijuana and alcohol.

After an apparently normal childhood, Mr. Evans began to show dysphoric mood, anhedonia, low energy, and social isolation by age 15. At about the same time, Mr. Ev-ans began to drink alcohol and smoke marijuana every day. In addition, he developed recurrent panic attacks, marked by a sudden onset of palpitations, diaphoresis, and thoughts that he was going to die. When he was at his most depressed and panicky, he twice received a combination of sertraline 100 mg/day and psychotherapy. In both cases, his most intense depressive symptoms lifted within a few weeks, and he dis-continued the sertraline after a few months. Between episodes of severe depression, he was generally seen as sad, irritable, and amotivated. His school performance de-clined around tenth grade and remained marginal through the rest of high school. He did not attend college as his parents had expected him to, but instead lived at home and did odd jobs in the neighborhood.

Around age 20, Mr. Evans developed a psychotic episode in which he had the con-viction that he had murdered people when he was 6 years old. Although he could not remember who these people were or the circumstances, he was absolutely convinced that this had happened, something that was confirmed by continuous voices accusing him of being a murderer. He also became convinced that other people would punish him for what had happened, and thus he feared for his life. Over the ensuing few weeks, he became guilt-ridden and preoccupied with the idea that he should kill him-self by slashing his wrists, which culminated in his being psychiatrically hospitalized. Although his affect on admission was anxious, within a couple of days he also became very depressed, with prominent anhedonia, poor sleep, and decreased appetite and concentration. With the combined use of antipsychotic and antidepressant medica-tions, both the depression and the psychotic symptoms remitted after 4 weeks. Thus, the total duration of the psychotic episode was approximately 7 weeks, 4 of which were also characterized by major depression. He was hospitalized with the same pat-tern of symptoms two additional times before age 22, each of which started with several weeks of delusions and hallucinations related to his conviction that he had murdered someone when he was a child, followed by severe depression lasting an additional month. Both relapses occurred while he was apparently adherent to reasonable dos-ages of antipsychotic and antidepressant medications. During the 3 years prior to this evaluation, Mr. Evans had been adherent to clozapine and had been without halluci-nations and delusions. He had also been adherent to his antidepressant medication and supportive psychotherapy, although his dysphoria, irritability, and amotivation never completely resolved.

Mr. Evans's history was significant for marijuana and alcohol abuse that began at age 15. Before the onset of psychosis at age 20, he smoked several joints of marijuana almost daily and binge drank on weekends, with occasional blackouts. After the onset of the psychosis, he decreased his marijuana and alcohol use significantly, with two several-month-long periods of abstinence, yet he continued to have psychotic episodes up through age 22. He started attending Alcoholics Anonymous and Narcotics Anonymous groups, achieved sobriety from marijuana and alcohol at age 23, and had remained sober for 2 years.

## Diagnoses

- Schizoaffective disorder, depressive type
- Alcohol use disorder, in remission
- Marijuana use disorder, in remission

## Discussion

Mr. Evans has struggled with depression and anxiety since adolescence, worsened by frequent use of marijuana and alcohol. At first, his treaters diagnosed him with depression and panic disorder and treated him accordingly. He did not enter college, as his family had expected, and he has not been employed since graduation from high school. At age 20, psychosis emerged and he required psychiatric hospitalization.

His major psychotic symptom is paranoia, with persecutory delusions and paramnesias of homicide. The delusions are worsened by auditory hallucinations, which he experiences as confirmation of his delusions. The delusions and hallucinations occurred almost daily between ages 20 and 22, until they resolved with clozapine treatment. Although he reports difficulties with his memory, he has not displayed marked cognitive impairment or disorganization of thought. He is socially isolated and minimally able to interact with others. The extent, severity, and duration of his psychotic symptoms are consistent with the diagnosis of a schizophrenia spectrum disorder.

Mr. Evans's psychosis emerged after several years of depression, anxiety, and panic attacks. Since the onset of his psychotic illness, he has experienced multiple episodes of depression, which emerge after periods of delusion and hallucinations and feature overwhelming guilt, prominent anhedonia, poor sleep, and occasional bursts of irritability. He can become suicidal when psychosis and depression reach peak intensity.

Mr. Evans meets criteria, therefore, for DSM-5 schizoaffective disorder. He has had an uninterrupted period in which his major depressive symptoms were concurrent with his schizophrenia symptoms. He has had several-week periods of hallucinations and delusions without prominent mood symptoms. Since the onset of the active and residual portions of his schizophrenia, the major depressive symptoms have been present most of the time.

Mr. Evans also used marijuana and alcohol for 8 years. Although these might have contributed to the emergence of his mood and psychotic symptoms, he continued to experience significant delusions, hallucinations, and depression between ages 20 and 22, when he stopped using marijuana and alcohol for several months. An alcohol- or marijuana-induced depressive, anxiety, or psychotic disorder might have been considered at various times in Mr. Evans's life, but the persistence of his mood and psychotic symptoms for months after the discontinuation of marijuana and alcohol indicates that he does not have a substance-induced psychiatric disorder.

His response to treatment with antipsychotic, antidepressant, and mood-stabilizing medication is typical: several failed attempts with antipsychotic drugs, the need for combined treatment during periods of exacerbations, and failed attempts to taper either the antidepressant or the antipsychotic medication.

One complicating factor in regard to diagnosing a DSM-5 schizoaffective disorder is the reality that although DSM-5 requires that the mood disorder be present for the majority of the active and residual portions of the schizophrenia, mood and psychotic disorders tend to vary significantly in regard to treatment response and clinical course. For example, whereas depressive and bipolar disorders tend to run in cycles, schizophrenia—once it unfolds—tends to persist. Furthermore, depressive and bipolar disorders tend to be more amenable to treatment than schizophrenia, especially because the diagnostic time frame for the latter includes the residual phase of schizophrenia, which can be largely resistant to psychiatric interventions. It remains to be seen how this tightening of the criteria for schizoaffective disorder will affect the identification and treatment of this cluster of patients.

## Suggested Reading

Heckers S: Diagnostic criteria for schizoaffective disorder. Expert Rev Neurother 12(1):1–3, 2012

# Case 6: Psychosis and Cannabis

*Melissa Nau, M.D.*
*Heather Warm, M.D.*

Kevin Foster, a 32-year-old white man with a history of bipolar disorder, was brought to the emergency room (ER) by police after his wife called 911 to report that he was threatening to jump out of their hotel window.

At the time of the episode, Mr. Foster and his wife were on vacation, celebrating their fifth anniversary. To commemorate the event, they decided to get tattoos. Afterward, they went to a nearby park, where Mr. Foster bought and smoked a marijuana cigarette. During the ensuing hour, Mr. Foster began to believe that the symbols in his tattoo had mysterious meaning and power. He became convinced that the tattoo artist was conspiring with others against him and that his wife was cheating on him. After returning to the hotel, the patient searched his wife's phone for evidence of her infidelity and threatened to jump out the window. The patient's wife, an ER physician, successfully convinced the patient to go to sleep, thinking that the episode would resolve.

The following day, the patient remained paranoid and delusional. He again threatened to jump out the window, and indicated that he would have no choice but to kill his wife the next time she slept. She called 911, and her husband was brought to the ER of a large nearby hospital. Later that day, he was admitted to an acute inpatient psychiatric unit with a diagnosis of unspecified psychotic disorder.

The patient had smoked cannabis sporadically from age 18 but began to smoke daily 5 years prior to this admission. He and his wife denied that he had ever used other illicit substances, and the patient indicated that he rarely drank alcohol. Until 1 year earlier, he had never seen a psychiatrist or been viewed by his friends and family as having significant psychiatric issues.

In the past year, however, Mr. Foster had been hospitalized four times for psychiatric problems. He had been hospitalized twice with classic manic symptoms and once for a suicidal depression. In addition, 7 months prior to this presentation, the patient had been hospitalized for a 6-week episode of cannabis-induced psychosis, which responded well to risperidone. At that time, his main symptom was paranoia. Two months prior to this admission, he entered a 1-month inpatient substance abuse treatment program for cannabis use disorder. Until the weekend of this admission, he had not used marijuana, alcohol, or any other substances since discharge from the rehabilitation facility. He had also been functioning well while taking lithium monotherapy for 3 months.

Mr. Foster had been steadily employed as a film editor since graduating from college. His father had a bipolar disorder, and his paternal grandfather committed suicide via gunshot but with an unknown diagnosis.

On the second day of hospitalization, the patient began to realize that his wife was not cheating on him and that the symbols in his tattoo were not meaningful. By the third day, he spontaneously said the paranoia was the result of cannabis intoxication. He declined further risperidone but continued lithium monotherapy. He was discharged with an appointment to follow up with his outpatient psychiatrist.

## Diagnoses

- Cannabis-induced psychotic disorder
- Bipolar disorder, in remission

## Discussion

Soon after smoking a marijuana cigarette, Mr. Foster began to believe that the symbols of his new tattoo had mysterious meaning and power. Within hours, he became paranoid about the tattoo artist and delusionally jealous. He threatened to kill himself and his wife. He was admitted to a psychiatric unit. The psychotic symptoms cleared within a few days, and the patient regained appropriate insight. This symptom trajectory fits DSM-5 substance/medication-induced psychotic disorder, which requires delusions or hallucinations that develop during, or soon after, a substance intoxication (or withdrawal or medication exposure).

An additional DSM-5 diagnostic criterion for cannabis-induced psychotic disorder revolves around whether Mr. Foster's delusions might not be better explained by a primary psychotic disorder such as schizophrenia or psychotic symptoms within depression or mania. His symptoms resolved within 3 days, which is typical for a cannabis-induced psychosis but not for an independent psychotic disorder. The rapid resolution of symptoms would support the likelihood that the cannabis caused his symptoms.

Mr. Foster's psychiatric history complicates the diagnosis in two different ways. First, of the four psychiatric hospitalizations Mr. Foster has had in the past year, one was for paranoid delusions in the context of cannabis use, leading to a 6-week hospitalization. The duration of the actual paranoid delusions is not entirely clear, but they appear to have lasted far longer than would be typical for a cannabis-induced psychosis. DSM-5 specifically cautions that persistence of a psychosis beyond 1 month after the exposure implies that the psychosis may be independent rather than substance induced.

Second, of Mr. Foster's three other psychiatric hospitalizations, two were for "classic" mania and one was for "suicidal depression." It is not clear whether paranoia or psychosis was part of these episodes. DSM-5 points out that a history of recurrent non-substance-related psychotic episodes would make a substance-induced psychosis less likely.

It is not clear whether these psychiatric episodes can be brought together under a single diagnostic umbrella. For example, Mr. Foster could have bipolar disorder with recurrent episodes of depression and mania. The cannabis might help him sleep— which might reduce the mania—but could possibly trigger episodes. If manic and depressive episodes (with or without psychosis) are triggered by a substance but symptoms persist for an extended period of time, then the most accurate diagnosis would be the bipolar disorder. This would be especially true if similar symptoms develop in the absence of substance use. Mr. Foster has a family history significant for bipolar disorder, which could further support such a diagnosis. On the other hand, Mr. Foster did not endorse any mood symptoms during this most recent psychotic episode, and psychotic symptoms resolved within 2–3 days. This history would seem to indicate that although Mr. Foster has historically met criteria for bipolar disorder, it seems to be currently in remission.

Multiple schizophrenia spectrum disorders might be considered. Given a 3-day duration of symptoms, however, most diagnoses are quickly eliminated as possibilities. In addition, Mr. Foster appears to have only one affected domain (delusions). Delusional disorder involves only delusions, but the minimum duration is 1 month. Brief psychotic disorder also requires only one of the four primary schizophrenia spectrum symptoms, but it does require an evaluation as to whether the precipitant might be a substance or medication.

At the moment, then, a cannabis-induced psychotic disorder appears to be the most likely diagnosis for Mr. Foster's particular episode. Clarification might be possible through more thorough investigation of prior medical records, but even more helpful will be ongoing, longitudinal follow-up.

## Suggested Readings

Caton CL, Hasin DS, Shrout PE, et al: Stability of early-phase primary psychotic disorders with concurrent substance use and substance-induced psychosis. Br J Psychiatry 190:105–111, 2007

Ekleberry S: Treating Co-Occurring Disorders: A Handbook for Mental Health and Substance Abuse Professionals. Binghamton, NY, Haworth, 2004

Grant BF, Stinson FS, Dawson DA, et al: Prevalence and co-occurrence of substance use disorders and independent mood and anxiety disorders: results from the National Epidemiologic Survey on Alcohol and Related Conditions. Arch Gen Psychiatry 61(8):807–816, 2004

Pettinati HM, O'Brien CP, Dundon WD: Current status of co-occurring mood and substance use disorders: a new therapeutic target. Am J Psychiatry 170(1):23–30, 2013

# Case 7: Flea Infestation

*Julie B. Penzner, M.D.*

Lara Gonzalez, a 51-year-old divorced freelance journalist, brought herself to the emergency room requesting dermatological evaluation for flea infestation. When no corroborating evidence was found on skin examination and the patient insisted that she was unsafe at home, she was admitted to an inpatient psychiatric service with "unspecified psychotic disorder."

Her concerns began around 1 week prior to presentation. To contend with financial stress, she had taken in temporary renters for a spare room in her home and had begun pet sitting for some neighbors. Under these conditions, she perceived brown insects burrowing into her skin and walls and covering her rugs and mattress. She threw away a bag of clothing, believing she heard fleas "rustling and scratching inside." She was not sleeping well, and she had spent the 36 hours prior to presentation frantically cleaning her home, fearing that her tenants would not pay if they saw the fleas. She showered multiple times using shampoos meant to treat animal infestations. She called an exterminator who found no evidence of fleas, but she did not believe him. She was upset about the infestation but was otherwise not troubled by depressive or manic symptoms, or by paranoia. She did not use drugs or alcohol. No one in the family had a history of psychiatric illness. Ms. Gonzalez had had depression once in the past and was briefly treated with an antidepressant. She had no relevant medical problems.

Her worries about infestation began in the setting of her sister's diagnosis with invasive cancer, the onset of her own menopause, financial strain that was likely forcing her to move from the United States back to Argentina (her country of origin), and a recent breakup with her boyfriend. At baseline, she described herself as an obsessive person who had always had contamination phobias, which historically worsened during times of anxiety.

On mental status examination, Ms. Gonzalez was calm and easily engaged, with normal relatedness and eye contact. She offered up a small plastic bag containing "fleas and larvae" that she had collected in the hospital while awaiting evaluation. Inspection of the bag revealed lint and plaster. Her speech had an urgent quality to it, and she described her mood as "sad right now." She was tearful intermittently but otherwise smiling reactively. Her thoughts were overly inclusive and intensely focused on fleas. She expressed belief that each time a hair fell out of her head, it would morph into larvae. When crying, she believed an egg came out of her tear duct. She was not suicidal or homicidal. She expressed an unshakable belief that lint was larvae, and that she was infested. She denied hallucinations. Cognition was intact. Her insight was impaired, but her judgment was deemed reasonably appropriate.

Dermatological examination revealed no insects or larvae embedded in Ms. Gonzalez's skin. Results of neurological examination, head computed tomography scan, laboratory tests, and toxicology data were normal. She was discharged on a low-dose antipsychotic medication and seen weekly for supportive psychotherapy. Her preoccupation improved within days and resolved entirely within 2 weeks. She developed enough insight to refer to her belief that fleas were in her skin as a "crazy thought." She attributed her "break from reality" to multiple stressors, and was able to articulate that she relied on her delusion as a way to distract herself from real problems. Her family corroborated her quick return to baseline.

## Diagnosis

- Brief psychotic disorder with marked stressors

## Discussion

Ms. Gonzalez's delusions with quick return to full premorbid functioning suggest a diagnosis of brief psychotic disorder with marked stressors. Formerly called "brief reactive psychosis," a brief psychotic disorder (with or without marked stressors) may not be diagnosed until return to baseline has occurred. The differential diagnosis of this condition is important.

At the time of admission, the patient was diagnosed with "unspecified psychotic disorder," a term often used when psychosis is present but information is incomplete. Only after her symptoms rapidly resolved could she be diagnosed with a brief psychotic disorder. Ms. Gonzalez's insight returned quite quickly, and she was able to link her symptoms to antecedent stressors. Although treatment is likely to shorten the duration of an acute psychotic episode, DSM-5 specifically does not factor treatment into the requirement that the episode last less than 1 month.

It is worth noting that stressors can be positive (e.g., marriage, new job, new baby) or negative, as in Ms. Gonzalez's case. A favorable prognosis is often associated with a history of good premorbid functioning, significant acute stressors, and a lack of family or personal history of psychiatric illness.

Ms. Gonzalez's sleeplessness, behavioral agitation, and premorbid depressive history might also suggest bipolar episode, but there are no other symptoms to support this diagnosis. Similarly, her delusional obsession with flea infestation suggests a possible delusional disorder, but Ms. Gonzalez's symptoms resolved far too quickly for this to be likely. Patients with personality disorders can have "micropsychoses," but Ms. Gonzalez does not appear to have a personality disorder or particular personality vulnerability. Malingering and factitious disorder appear unlikely, as do delirium and other medically mediated illnesses.

Brief psychotic episodes have a low prevalence in the population, which could indicate that brief psychoses are unusual. It could also indicate that people with a very short duration of psychotic symptoms may not seek psychiatric help. The brevity and unpredictability of symptoms also makes it difficult to do research and for any particular clinician or institution to develop an expertise. Brief psychotic episodes are also noted to have a relatively low stability over time, which makes sense given that—unlike schizophrenia—brief psychotic episodes are, by definition, of short duration and cannot even be diagnosed without both remission of symptoms and careful follow-up.

## Suggested Readings

Jørgensen P, Bennedsen B, Christensen J, et al: Acute and transient psychotic disorder: comorbidity with personality disorder. Acta Psychiatr Scand 94(6):460–464, 1996

Salvatore P, Baldessarini RJ, Tohen M, et al: McLean-Harvard International First-Episode Project: two-year stability of DSM-IV diagnoses in 500 first-episode psychotic disorder patients. J Clin Psychiatry 70(4):458–466, 2009

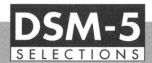
1. Criterion A for schizoaffective disorder requires an uninterrupted period of illness during which Criterion A for schizophrenia is met. Which of the following additional symptoms must be present to fulfill diagnostic criteria for schizoaffective disorder?

   A. An anxiety episode—either panic or general anxiety.
   B. Rapid eye movement (REM) sleep behavior disorder.
   C. A major depressive or manic episode.
   D. Hypomania.
   E. Cyclothymia.

2. There is a requirement for a major depressive episode or a manic episode to be part of the symptom picture for a DSM-5 diagnosis of schizoaffective disorder. In order to separate schizoaffective disorder from depressive or bipolar disorder with psychotic features, which of the following symptoms must be present for at least 2 weeks in the absence of a major mood episode at some point during the lifetime duration of the illness?

   A. Delusions or hallucinations.
   B. Delusions or paranoia.
   C. Regressed behavior.
   D. Projective identification.
   E. Binge eating.

3. A 27-year-old unmarried truck driver has a 5-year history of active and residual symptoms of schizophrenia. He develops symptoms of depression, including depressed mood and anhedonia, that last 4 months and resolve with treatment but do not meet criteria for major depression. Which diagnosis best fits this clinical presentation?

   A. Schizoaffective disorder.
   B. Unspecified schizophrenia spectrum and other psychotic disorder.
   C. Unspecified depressive disorder.
   D. Schizophrenia and unspecified depressive disorder.
   E. Unspecified bipolar and related disorder.

4.  How common is schizoaffective disorder relative to schizophrenia?

    A. Much more common.
    B. Twice as common.
    C. Equally common.
    D. One-half as common.
    E. One-third as common.

5.  A 30-year-old single woman reports having experienced auditory and perse-cutory delusions for 2 months, followed by a full major depressive episode with sad mood, anhedonia, and suicidal ideation lasting 3 months. Although the depressive episode resolves with pharmacotherapy and psychotherapy, the psychotic symptoms persist for another month before resolving. What di-agnosis best fits this clinical picture?

    A. Brief psychotic disorder.
    B. Schizoaffective disorder.
    C. Major depressive disorder.
    D. Major depressive disorder with psychotic features.
    E. Bipolar I disorder, current episode manic, with mixed features.

6.  Which of the following statements about the incidence of schizoaffective disor-der is *true?*

    A. The incidence is equal in women and men.
    B. The incidence is higher in men.
    C. The incidence is higher in women.
    D. The incidence rates are unknown.
    E. The incidence rates vary based on seasonality of birth.

7.  Substance/medication-induced psychotic disorder cannot be diagnosed if the disturbance is better explained by an independent psychotic disorder that is not induced by a substance/medication. Which of the following psychotic symp-tom presentations would *not* be evidence of an independent psychotic disorder?

    A. Psychotic symptoms that precede the onset of severe intoxication or acute withdrawal.
    B. Psychotic symptoms that meet full criteria for a psychotic disorder and that persist for a substantial period after cessation of severe intoxication or acute withdrawal.
    C. Psychotic symptoms that are substantially in excess of what would be ex-pected given the type or amount of the substance used or the duration of use.
    D. Psychotic symptoms that occur during a period of sustained substance ab-stinence.
    E. Psychotic symptoms that occur during a medical admission for substance withdrawal.

8.   A 55-year-old man with a known history of alcohol dependence and schizo-phrenia is brought to the emergency department because of frank delusions and visual hallucinations. Which of the following would *not* be a diagnostic possibility for inclusion in the differential diagnosis?

A.  Schizophrenia.
B.  Substance/medication-induced psychotic disorder.
C.  Alcohol dependence.
D.  Psychotic disorder due to another medical condition.
E.  Borderline personality disorder with psychotic features.

9.   Which of the following sets of specifiers is included in the DSM-5 diagnostic criteria for substance/medication-induced psychotic disorder?

A.  "With onset before intoxication" and "With onset before withdrawal."
B.  "With onset during intoxication" and "With onset during withdrawal."
C.  "With good prognostic features" and "Without good prognostic features."
D.  "With onset prior to substance use" and "With onset after substance use."
E.  "With catatonia" and 'Without catatonia."

10.  A 65-year-old man with systemic lupus erythematosus who is being treated with corticosteroids witnesses a serious motor vehicle accident. He begins to have disorganized speech, which lasts for several days before resolving. What diagnosis best fits this clinical picture?

A.  Schizophrenia.
B.  Psychotic disorder associated with systemic lupus erythematosus.
C.  Steroid-induced psychosis.
D.  Brief psychotic disorder, with marked stressor.
E.  Schizoaffective disorder.

11.  Which of the following psychotic symptom presentations would *not* be appro-priately diagnosed as "other specified schizophrenia spectrum and other psy-chotic disorder"?

A.  Psychotic symptoms that have lasted for less than 1 month but have not yet remitted, so that the criteria for brief psychotic disorder are not met.
B.  Persistent auditory hallucinations occurring in the absence of any other fea-tures.
C.  Postpartum psychosis that does not meet criteria for a depressive or bipolar disorder with psychotic features, brief psychotic disorder, psychotic disorder due to another medical condition, or substance/medication-induced psy-chotic disorder.
D.  Psychotic symptoms that are temporally related to use of a substance.
E.  Persistent delusions with periods of overlapping mood episodes that are present for a substantial portion of the delusional disturbance.

12. Which of the following patient presentations would *not* be classified as psychotic for the purpose of diagnosing schizophrenia?

    A. A patient is hearing a voice that tells him he is a special person.
    B. A patient believes he is being followed by a secret police organization that is focused exclusively on him.
    C. A patient has a flashback to a war experience that feels like it is happening again.
    D. A patient cannot organize his thoughts and stops responding in the middle of an interview.
    E. A patient presents wearing an automobile tire around his waist and gives no explanation.

13. In which of the following disorders can psychotic symptoms occur?

    A. Bipolar and depressive disorders.
    B. Substance use disorders.
    C. Posttraumatic stress disorder.
    D. Other medical conditions.
    E. All of the above.

14. A 32-year-old man presents to the emergency department distressed and agitated. He reports that his sister has been killed in a car accident on a trip to South America. When asked how he found out, he says that he and his sister were very close and he "just knows it." After putting him on the phone with his sister, who was comfortably staying with friends while on her trip, the man expressed relief that she was alive. Which of the following descriptions best fits this presentation?

    A. He had a delusional belief, because he believed it was true without good warrant.
    B. He did not have a delusional belief, because it changed in light of new evidence.
    C. He had a grandiose delusion, because he believed he could know things happening far away.
    D. He had a nihilistic delusion, because it involved an untrue, imagined catastrophe.
    E. He did not have a delusion, because in some cultures people believe they can know things about family members outside of ordinary communications.

15. Which of the following is *not* a commonly recognized type of delusion?

    A. Persecutory.
    B. Erotomanic.
    C. Alien abduction.

D. Somatic.

E. Grandiose.

16. A 64-year-old man who had been a widower for 3 months presents to the emergency department on the advice of his primary care physician after he reports to the doctor that he hears his deceased wife's voice calling his name when he looks through old photos, and sometimes as he is trying to fall asleep. His primary care physician tells him he is having a psychotic episode and needs to get a psychiatric evaluation. Which of the following statements correctly explains why these experiences are not considered to be psychotic?

    A. The voice he hears is from a family member.

    B. The experience occurs as he is falling asleep.

    C. He can invoke her voice with certain activities.

    D. The voice calls his name.

    E. Both B and C.

17. A 19-year-old college student is brought by ambulance to the emergency department. His college dorm supervisor, who called the ambulance, reports that the student was isolating himself, was pacing in his room, and was not responding to questions. In the emergency department, the patient gets down in a crouching position and begins making barking noises at seemingly random times. His urine toxicology report is negative, and all labs are within normal limits. What is the best description of these symptoms?

    A. An animal delusion—the patient believes he is a dog.

    B. Intermittent explosive rage.

    C. A paranoid stance leading to self-protective aggression.

    D. Catatonic behavior.

    E. Formal thought disorder.

18. Which of the following does *not* represent a negative symptom of schizophrenia?

    A. Affective flattening.

    B. Decreased motivation.

    C. Impoverished thought processes.

    D. Sadness over loss of functionality.

    E. Social disinterest.

19. Schizophrenia spectrum and other psychotic disorders are defined by abnormalities in one or more of five domains, four of which are also considered psychotic symptoms. Which of the following is *not* considered a psychotic symptom?

    A. Delusions.

    B. Hallucinations.

    C. Disorganized thinking.

      D. Disorganized or abnormal motor behavior.

      E. Avolition.

20.     What is the most common type of delusion?

      A. Somatic delusion of distorted body appearance.

      B. Grandiose delusion.

      C. Thought insertion.

      D. Persecutory delusion.

      E. Former life regression.

21.     Label each of the following beliefs as a bizarre delusion, a nonbizarre delusion, or a nondelusion.

      A. A 25-year-old law student believes he has uncovered the truth about JFK's assassination and that CIA agents have been dispatched to follow him and monitor his Internet communications.

      B. A 45-year-old homeless man presents to the psychiatric emergency room complaining of a skin rash. Upon removal of his clothes, it is seen that most of his body is wrapped in aluminum foil. The man explains that he is protecting himself from the electromagnetic ray guns that are constantly targeting him.

      C. A 47-year-old unemployed plumber believes he has been elected to the House of Representatives. When the Capitol police evict him and bring him to the emergency department, he says that they are Tea Party activists who are merely impersonating police officers.

      D. A 35-year-old high school physics teacher presents to your office with insomnia and tells you that he has discovered and memorized the formula for cold fusion energy, only to have the formula removed from his memory by telepathic aliens.

      E. An 18-year-old recent immigrant from Eastern Europe believes that wearing certain colors will ward off the "evil eye" and prevent catastrophes that would otherwise occur.

22.     Which of the following presentations would *not* be classified as disorganized behavior for the purpose of diagnosing schizophrenia spectrum and other psychotic disorders?

      A. Masturbating in public.

      B. Wearing slacks on one's head.

      C. Responding verbally to auditory hallucinations in a conversational mode.

      D. Crouching on all fours and barking.

      E. Turning to face 180 degrees away from the interviewer when answering questions.

23. Which of the following statements about catatonic motor behaviors is *false?*

    A. Catatonic motor behavior is a type of grossly disorganized behavior that has historically been associated with schizophrenia spectrum and other psychotic disorders.
    B. Catatonic motor behaviors may occur in many mental disorders (such as mood disorders) and in other medical conditions.
    C. A behavior is considered catatonic only if it involves motoric slowing or rigidity, such as mutism, posturing, or waxy flexibility.
    D. Catatonia can be diagnosed independently of another psychiatric disorder.
    E. Catatonic behaviors involve markedly reduced reactivity to the environment.

24. Which of the following statements about negative symptoms of schizophrenia is *false?*

    A. Negative symptoms are easily distinguished from medication side effects such as sedation.
    B. Negative symptoms include diminished emotional expression.
    C. Negative symptoms can be difficult to distinguish from medication side effects such as sedation.
    D. Negative symptoms include reduced peer or social interaction.
    E. Negative symptoms include decreased motivation for goal-directed activities.

25. Which of the following statements correctly describes a way in which schizoaffective disorder may be differentiated from bipolar disorder?

    A. Schizoaffective disorder involves only depressive episodes, never manic or hypomanic episodes.
    B. In bipolar disorder, psychotic symptoms do not last longer than 1 month.
    C. In bipolar disorder, psychotic symptoms are always cotemporal with mood symptoms.
    D. Schizoaffective disorder never includes full-blown episodes of major depression.
    E. In bipolar disorder, psychotic symptoms are always mood congruent.

26. Which of the following symptom combinations, if present for 1 month, would meet Criterion A for schizophrenia?

    A. Prominent auditory and visual hallucinations.
    B. Grossly disorganized behavior and avolition.
    C. Disorganized speech and diminished emotional expression.
    D. Paranoid and grandiose delusions.
    E. Avolition and diminished emotional expression.

27.    Which of the following statements about violent or suicidal behavior in schizophrenia is *false?*

A.  About 5%–6% of individuals with schizophrenia die by suicide.
B.  Persons with schizophrenia frequently assault strangers in a random fashion.
C.  Compared with the general population, persons with schizophrenia are more frequently victims of violence.
D.  Command hallucinations to harm oneself sometimes precede suicidal behaviors.
E.  Youth, male gender, and substance abuse are factors that increase the risk for suicide among persons with schizophrenia.

28.    Which of the following statements about childhood-onset schizophrenia is *true?*

A.  Childhood-onset schizophrenia tends to resemble poor-outcome adult schizophrenia, with gradual onset and prominent negative symptoms.
B.  Disorganized speech patterns in childhood are usually indicative of schizophrenia.
C.  Because of the childhood capacity for imagination, delusions and hallucinations in childhood-onset schizophrenia are more elaborate than those in adult-onset schizophrenia.
D.  In a child presenting with disorganized behavior, schizophrenia should be ruled out before other childhood diagnoses are considered.
E.  Visual hallucinations are extremely rare in childhood-onset schizophrenia.

29.    Which of the following statements about gender differences in schizophrenia is *true?*

A.  Women with schizophrenia tend to have fewer psychotic symptoms than do men over the course of the illness.
B.  A first onset of schizophrenia after age 40 is more likely in women than in men.
C.  Psychotic symptoms in women tend to burn out with age to a greater extent than they do in men.
D.  Negative symptoms and affective flattening are more frequently observed in women with schizophrenia than in men with the disorder.
E.  The overall incidence of schizophrenia is higher in women than it is in men.

30.    A 19-year-old female college student is brought to the emergency department by her family over her objections. Three months ago, she suddenly started feeling "odd," and she came home from college because she could not concentrate. Two weeks after she came home, she began hearing voices telling her that she is "a sinner" and must repent. Although never a religious person, she now believes she must repent, but she does not know how, and feels confused. She is managing her activities of daily living despite the ongoing auditory hallucinations and delusions, and she is affectively reactive on examination. Which diagnosis best fits this presentation?

    A. Schizophreniform disorder, with good prognostic features, provisional.
    B. Schizophreniform disorder, without good prognostic features, provisional.
    C. Schizophreniform disorder, with good prognostic features.
    D. Schizophreniform disorder, without good prognostic features.
    E. Unspecified schizophrenia spectrum and other psychotic disorder.

31. A 24-year-old male college student is brought to the emergency department by the college health service team. A few weeks ago he was involved in a car accident in which one of his friends was critically injured and died in his arms. The man has not come out of his room or showered for the last 2 weeks. He has eaten only minimally, claimed that aliens have targeted him for abduction, and asserted that he could hear their radio transmissions. Nothing seems to convince him that this abduction will not happen or that the transmissions are not real. Which of the following diagnoses (and justifications) is most appropriate for this man?

    A. Brief psychotic disorder with a marked stressor, because the symptoms began after the tragic car accident.
    B. Brief psychotic disorder without a marked stressor, because the content of the psychosis is unrelated to the accident.
    C. Unspecified schizophrenia spectrum and other psychotic disorder, because more information is needed.
    D. Schizophreniform disorder, because there are psychotic symptoms but not yet a full-blown schizophrenia picture.
    E. Delusional disorder, because the central symptom is a delusion of persecution.

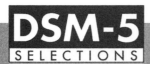

# Schizophrenia Spectrum and Other Psychotic Disorders

## DSM-5® Self-Exam Answer Guide

1. Criterion A for schizoaffective disorder requires an uninterrupted period of illness during which Criterion A for schizophrenia is met. Which of the following additional symptoms must be present to fulfill diagnostic criteria for schizoaffective disorder?

   A. An anxiety episode—either panic or general anxiety.
   B. Rapid eye movement (REM) sleep behavior disorder.
   C. A major depressive or manic episode.
   D. Hypomania.
   E. Cyclothymia.

   **Correct Answer: C. A major depressive or manic episode.**

   **Explanation:** The diagnosis of schizoaffective disorder is based on the presence of an uninterrupted period of illness during which Criterion A for schizophrenia is met. Criterion B (social dysfunction) and Criterion F (exclusion of autism spectrum disorder or other communication disorder of childhood onset) for schizophrenia do not have to be met. In addition to meeting Criterion A for schizophrenia, there must be a major mood episode (major depressive or manic) (Criterion A for schizoaffective disorder). Because loss of interest or pleasure is common in schizophrenia, to meet Criterion A for schizoaffective disorder, the major depressive episode must include pervasive depressed mood (i.e., the presence of markedly diminished interest or pleasure is not sufficient). The episodes of depression or mania must be present for the majority of the total duration of the illness (i.e., after Criterion A has been met) (Criterion C for schizoaffective disorder).

   1—Schizoaffective Disorder / Diagnostic Features (pp. 106–107)

2. There is a requirement for a major depressive episode or a manic episode to be part of the symptom picture for a DSM-5 diagnosis of schizoaffective disorder. In order to separate schizoaffective disorder from depressive or bipolar disorder with psychotic features, which of the following symptoms must be present for at least 2 weeks in the absence of a major mood episode at some point during the lifetime duration of the illness?

A. Delusions or hallucinations.
B. Delusions or paranoia.
C. Regressed behavior.
D. Projective identification.
E. Binge eating.

**Correct Answer: A. Delusions or hallucinations.**

**Explanation:** To separate schizoaffective disorder from a depressive or bipolar disorder with psychotic features, Criterion B for schizoaffective disorder specifies that delusions or hallucinations must be present for at least 2 weeks in the absence of a major mood episode (depressive or manic) at some point during the lifetime duration of the illness.

**2—Schizoaffective Disorder / Diagnostic Features (pp. 106–107)**

3. A 27-year-old unmarried truck driver has a 5-year history of active and residual symptoms of schizophrenia. He develops symptoms of depression, including depressed mood and anhedonia, that last 4 months and resolve with treatment but do not meet criteria for major depression. Which diagnosis best fits this clinical presentation?

   A. Schizoaffective disorder.
   B. Unspecified schizophrenia spectrum and other psychotic disorder.
   C. Unspecified depressive disorder.
   D. Schizophrenia and unspecified depressive disorder.
   E. Unspecified bipolar and related disorder.

**Correct Answer: D. Schizophrenia and unspecified depressive disorder.**

**Explanation:** The depressive and manic episodes, taken together, do not occupy more than 1 year during the 5-year history. Thus, the presentation does not meet Criterion C for schizoaffective disorder, and the diagnosis remains schizophrenia. The additional diagnosis of unspecified depressive disorder may be added to indicate the superimposed depressive episode.

**3—Schizoaffective Disorder / Differential Diagnosis (pp. 109–110)**

4. How common is schizoaffective disorder relative to schizophrenia?

   A. Much more common.
   B. Twice as common.
   C. Equally common.
   D. One-half as common.
   E. One-third as common.

**Correct Answer: E. One-third as common.**

**Explanation:** Schizoaffective disorder appears to be about one-third as common as schizophrenia, with a lifetime prevalence of 0.3%.

**4—Schizoaffective Disorder / Prevalence (pp. 107–108)**

5. A 30-year-old single woman reports having experienced auditory and persecutory delusions for 2 months, followed by a full major depressive episode with sad mood, anhedonia, and suicidal ideation lasting 3 months. Although the depressive episode resolves with pharmacotherapy and psychotherapy, the psychotic symptoms persist for another month before resolving. What diagnosis best fits this clinical picture?

   A. Brief psychotic disorder.
   B. Schizoaffective disorder.
   C. Major depressive disorder.
   D. Major depressive disorder with psychotic features.
   E. Bipolar I disorder, current episode manic, with mixed features.

**Correct Answer: B. Schizoaffective disorder.**

**Explanation:** During this period of illness, the woman's symptoms concurrently met criteria for a major depressive episode and Criterion A for schizophrenia. Auditory hallucinations and delusions were present both before and after the depressive phase. The total period of illness lasted for about 6 months, with psychotic symptoms alone present during the initial 2 months, both depressive and psychotic symptoms present during the next 3 months, and psychotic symptoms alone present during the last month. The duration of the depressive episode was not brief relative to the total duration of the psychotic disturbance.

**5—Schizoaffective Disorder / Diagnostic Features (pp. 106–107); Differential Diagnosis (pp. 109–110)**

6. Which of the following statements about the incidence of schizoaffective disorder is *true?*

   A. The incidence is equal in women and men.
   B. The incidence is higher in men.
   C. The incidence is higher in women.
   D. The incidence rates are unknown.
   E. The incidence rates vary based on seasonality of birth.

**Correct Answer: C. The incidence is higher in women.**

**Explanation:** The incidence of schizoaffective disorder is higher in women than in men, mainly due to an increased incidence of the depressive type among women.

**6—Schizoaffective Disorder / Prevalence (pp. 107–108)**

7. Substance/medication-induced psychotic disorder cannot be diagnosed if the disturbance is better explained by an independent psychotic disorder that is not induced by a substance/medication. Which of the following psychotic symptom presentations would *not* be evidence of an independent psychotic disorder?

A. Psychotic symptoms that precede the onset of severe intoxication or acute withdrawal.
B. Psychotic symptoms that meet full criteria for a psychotic disorder and that persist for a substantial period after cessation of severe intoxication or acute withdrawal.
C. Psychotic symptoms that are substantially in excess of what would be expected given the type or amount of the substance used or the duration of use.
D. Psychotic symptoms that occur during a period of sustained substance abstinence.
E. Psychotic symptoms that occur during a medical admission for substance withdrawal.

**Correct Answer: E. Psychotic symptoms that occur during a medical admission for substance withdrawal.**

**Explanation:** A substance/medication-induced psychotic disorder is distinguished from a primary psychotic disorder by considering the onset, course, and other factors. For drugs of abuse, there must be evidence from the history, physical examination, or laboratory findings of substance use, intoxication, or withdrawal. Substance/medication-induced psychotic disorders arise during or soon after exposure to a medication or after substance intoxication or withdrawal but can persist for weeks, whereas primary psychotic disorders may precede the onset of substance/medication use or may occur during times of sustained abstinence. Once initiated, the psychotic symptoms may continue as long as the substance/medication use continues. Another consideration is the presence of features that are atypical of a primary psychotic disorder (e.g., atypical age at onset or course). For example, the appearance of delusions de novo in a person older than 35 years without a known history of a primary psychotic disorder should suggest the possibility of a substance/medication-induced psychotic disorder. Even a prior history of a primary psychotic disorder does not rule out the possibility of a substance/medication-induced psychotic disorder. In contrast, factors that suggest that the psychotic symptoms are better accounted for by a primary psychotic disorder include persistence of psychotic symptoms for a substantial period of time (i.e., a month or more) after the end of substance intoxication or acute substance withdrawal or after cessation of medication use; or a history of prior recurrent primary psychotic disorders. Other causes of psychotic symptoms must be considered even in an individual with substance intoxication or withdrawal, because substance use problems are not uncommon among individuals with non-substance/medication-induced psychotic disorders.

7—Substance/Medication-Induced Psychotic Disorder / Diagnostic Features (pp. 112–113)

8.  A 55-year-old man with a known history of alcohol dependence and schizophrenia is brought to the emergency department because of frank delusions and visual hallucinations. Which of the following would *not* be a diagnostic possibility for inclusion in the differential diagnosis?

    A. Schizophrenia.
    B. Substance/medication-induced psychotic disorder.
    C. Alcohol dependence.
    D. Psychotic disorder due to another medical condition.
    E. Borderline personality disorder with psychotic features.

    **Correct Answer: E. Borderline personality disorder with psychotic features.**

    **Explanation:** There is no evidence provided for a diagnosis of borderline personality disorder. A prior history of a primary psychotic disorder (schizophrenia) does not rule out the possibility of a substance/medication-induced psychotic disorder. The appearance of delusions de novo in a person older than 35 years without a known history of primary psychotic disorder should suggest the possibility of a substance/medication-induced psychotic disorder.

    8—Substance/Medication-Induced Psychotic Disorder / Differential Diagnosis (pp. 109–110)

9.  Which of the following sets of specifiers is included in the DSM-5 diagnostic criteria for substance/medication-induced psychotic disorder?

    A. "With onset before intoxication" and "With onset before withdrawal."
    B. "With onset during intoxication" and "With onset during withdrawal."
    C. "With good prognostic features" and "Without good prognostic features."
    D. "With onset prior to substance use" and "With onset after substance use."
    E. "With catatonia" and 'Without catatonia."

    **Correct Answer: B. "With onset during intoxication" and "With onset during withdrawal."**

    **Explanation:** The specifier "with onset during intoxication" should be used if criteria for intoxication with the substance are met and the symptoms develop during intoxication. The specifier "with onset during withdrawal" should be used if criteria for withdrawal from the substance are met and the symptoms develop during, or shortly after, withdrawal.

    9—Substance/Medication-Induced Psychotic Disorder / diagnostic criteria (pp. 111–112)

10. A 65-year-old man with systemic lupus erythematosus who is being treated with corticosteroids witnesses a serious motor vehicle accident. He begins to have disorganized speech, which lasts for several days before resolving. What diagnosis best fits this clinical picture?

   A. Schizophrenia.
   B. Psychotic disorder associated with systemic lupus erythematosus.
   C. Steroid-induced psychosis.
   D. Brief psychotic disorder, with marked stressor.
   E. Schizoaffective disorder.

**Correct Answer: D. Brief psychotic disorder, with marked stressor.**

**Explanation:** The essential features of psychotic disorder due to another medical condition are prominent delusions or hallucinations that are judged to be attributable to the physiological effects of another medical condition and are not better explained by another mental disorder (e.g., the symptoms are not a psychologically mediated response to a severe medical condition, in which case a diagnosis of brief psychotic disorder, with marked stressor, would be appropriate). In the vignette above, the symptoms are better understood as being a psychologically mediated response to the trauma of witnessing the accident.

**10—Psychotic Disorder Due to Another Medical Condition / Diagnostic Features (p. 116)**

11. Which of the following psychotic symptom presentations would *not* be appropriately diagnosed as "other specified schizophrenia spectrum and other psychotic disorder"?

   A. Psychotic symptoms that have lasted for less than 1 month but have not yet remitted, so that the criteria for brief psychotic disorder are not met.
   B. Persistent auditory hallucinations occurring in the absence of any other features.
   C. Postpartum psychosis that does not meet criteria for a depressive or bipolar disorder with psychotic features, brief psychotic disorder, psychotic disorder due to another medical condition, or substance/medication-induced psychotic disorder.
   D. Psychotic symptoms that are temporally related to use of a substance.
   E. Persistent delusions with periods of overlapping mood episodes that are present for a substantial portion of the delusional disturbance.

**Correct Answer: D. Psychotic symptoms that are temporally related to use of a substance.**

**Explanation:** Psychotic symptoms that are temporally related to use of a substance would likely meet criteria for a DSM-5 substance/medication-induced psychotic disorder. The category *other specified schizophrenia spectrum and other psychotic disorder* applies to presentations in which symptoms characteristic of a schizophrenia spectrum and other psychotic disorder that cause clinically significant distress or impairment in social, occupational, or other important areas of functioning predominate but do not meet the full criteria for any of the disorders in the schizophrenia spectrum and other psychotic disorders diagnostic class. The other specified schizophrenia spectrum and other psychotic disorder category is used in situations in which the clinician chooses to communicate the specific reason that the presentation does not meet the criteria for any specific schizophrenia spectrum and other psychotic disorder. This is done by recording "other specified schizophrenia spectrum and other psychotic disorder" followed by the specific reason (e.g., "persistent auditory hallucinations").

**11—Other Specified Schizophrenia Spectrum and Other Psychotic Disorder (p. 122)**

12. Which of the following patient presentations would *not* be classified as psychotic for the purpose of diagnosing schizophrenia?

    A. A patient is hearing a voice that tells him he is a special person.
    B. A patient believes he is being followed by a secret police organization that is focused exclusively on him.
    C. A patient has a flashback to a war experience that feels like it is happening again.
    D. A patient cannot organize his thoughts and stops responding in the middle of an interview.
    E. A patient presents wearing an automobile tire around his waist and gives no explanation.

    **Correct Answer: C. A patient has a flashback to a war experience that feels like it is happening again.**

    **Explanation:** Schizophrenia spectrum and other psychotic disorders are defined by abnormalities in one or more of the following five domains, the first four of which are considered to be psychotic symptoms: delusions, hallucinations, disorganized thinking (speech), grossly disorganized or abnormal motor behavior (including catatonia), and negative symptoms. A flashback to a traumatic experience is an intense, emotionally laden memory but does not reach the level of a psychotic symptom.

    **12—chapter intro; Key Features That Define the Psychotic Disorders (pp. 87–88)**

13. In which of the following disorders can psychotic symptoms occur?

    A. Bipolar and depressive disorders.
    B. Substance use disorders.
    C. Posttraumatic stress disorder.
    D. Other medical conditions.
    E. All of the above.

**Correct Answer: E. All of the above.**

**Explanation:** Mood disorders, substance use disorders, posttraumatic stress disorder, and other medical conditions all can include psychotic symptoms as part of their presentation. Thus, clinicians must consider these and other possibilities before concluding that a patient's psychosis to due to a primary psychotic disorder.

**13—Brief Psychotic Disorder; Schizophrenia / Differential Diagnosis (pp. 96, 104–105)**

14. A 32-year-old man presents to the emergency department distressed and agitated. He reports that his sister has been killed in a car accident on a trip to South America. When asked how he found out, he says that he and his sister were very close and he "just knows it." After putting him on the phone with his sister, who was comfortably staying with friends while on her trip, the man expressed relief that she was alive. Which of the following descriptions best fits this presentation?

    A. He had a delusional belief, because he believed it was true without good warrant.
    B. He did not have a delusional belief, because it changed in light of new evidence.
    C. He had a grandiose delusion, because he believed he could know things happening far away.
    D. He had a nihilistic delusion, because it involved an untrue, imagined catastrophe.
    E. He did not have a delusion, because in some cultures people believe they can know things about family members outside of ordinary communications.

**Correct Answer: B. He did not have a delusional belief, because it changed in light of new evidence.**

**Explanation:** To be a delusion, a belief must be clearly false and must be fixed—that is, not amenable to change in light of additional information. This man's belief was false but held flexibly, and it was conditional on the evidence, such as talking to his living sister. Thus, it is not a delusion. Although cultural factors should be taken into account in determining whether a belief is delusional, that consideration is not relevant here, because the belief is not delusional independent of cultural background.

**14—Key Features That Define the Psychotic Disorders / Delusions (p. 87)**

15. Which of the following is *not* a commonly recognized type of delusion?

    A. Persecutory.
    B. Erotomanic.
    C. Alien abduction.

D. Somatic.

E. Grandiose.

**Correct Answer: C. Alien abduction.**

**Explanation:** Commonly recognized delusion types include persecutory, referential, somatic, nihilistic, grandiose and erotomanic, as well as combinations of these types. A delusional belief in alien abduction may be grandiose and may involve somatic and/or erotomanic aspects, but it is not itself a major category of delusional thought.

**15—Key Features That Define the Psychotic Disorders / Delusions (p. 87)**

16. A 64-year-old man who had been a widower for 3 months presents to the emergency department on the advice of his primary care physician after he reports to the doctor that he hears his deceased wife's voice calling his name when he looks through old photos, and sometimes as he is trying to fall asleep. His primary care physician tells him he is having a psychotic episode and needs to get a psychiatric evaluation. Which of the following statements correctly explains why these experiences are not considered to be psychotic?

    A. The voice he hears is from a family member.
    B. The experience occurs as he is falling asleep.
    C. He can invoke her voice with certain activities.
    D. The voice calls his name.
    E. Both B and C.

**Correct Answer: E. Both B and C.**

**Explanation:** If an auditory experience occurs only secondary to a controllable action (such as looking through highly affectively charged photos) or in an altered sensorial state, such as just before falling asleep (*hypnagogic*) or just as one is waking up (*hypnopompic*), it is not classified as a hallucination. Frank auditory hallucinations can involve the voice of someone known to the patient and often includes hearing one's name called.

**16—Key Features That Define the Psychotic Disorders / Hallucinations (pp. 87–88)**

17. A 19-year-old college student is brought by ambulance to the emergency department. His college dorm supervisor, who called the ambulance, reports that the student was isolating himself, was pacing in his room, and was not responding to questions. In the emergency department, the patient gets down in a crouching position and begins making barking noises at seemingly random times. His urine toxicology report is negative, and all labs are within normal limits. What is the best description of these symptoms?

    A. An animal delusion—the patient believes he is a dog.
    B. Intermittent explosive rage.

    C. A paranoid stance leading to self-protective aggression.
    D. Catatonic behavior.
    E. Formal thought disorder.

**Correct Answer: D. Catatonic behavior.**

**Explanation:** Delusions involve beliefs, but we cannot assess the patient's belief structure or his formal thought patterns since he is not answering questions. Similarly, rage is an emotion that may result in intense motor activity, but we have not been able to assess the patient's thought content or his emotions. The patient is likely exhibiting psychomotor agitation but it is of a specific type, namely catatonic excitement that does not relate to the environment or to any goal-directed motivation. Mutism followed by catatonic excitement, such as stereotypic vocalizations, can occur in catatonia.

    **17—Key Features That Define the Psychotic Disorders / Grossly Disorganized or Abnormal Motor Behavior (Including Catatonia) (p. 88)**

18. Which of the following does *not* represent a negative symptom of schizophrenia?

    A. Affective flattening.
    B. Decreased motivation.
    C. Impoverished thought processes.
    D. Sadness over loss of functionality.
    E. Social disinterest.

**Correct Answer: D. Sadness over loss of functionality.**

**Explanation:** Patients with schizophrenia may be aware of their functional losses and may feel sadness about this. That emotional response would be the opposite of negative symptoms, because it would involve an active and expressive-emotional response. The other symptoms mentioned—affective flattening, decreased motivation, impoverished thought process, and social disinterest—are all part of the negative or deficit symptoms of schizophrenia. It is thus important to distinguish the uses of the word "negative." In reference to sad emotions it has one meaning, but the "negative" symptoms of schizophrenia mean deficits of normal psychological functioning, including absence of sad feelings.

    **18—Key Features That Define the Psychotic Disorders / Negative Symptoms (p. 88)**

19. Schizophrenia spectrum and other psychotic disorders are defined by abnormalities in one or more of five domains, four of which are also considered psychotic symptoms. Which of the following is *not* considered a psychotic symptom?

    A. Delusions.
    B. Hallucinations.

C. Disorganized thinking.
D. Disorganized or abnormal motor behavior.
E. Avolition.

**Correct Answer: E. Avolition.**

**Explanation:** Avolition is a negative symptom of schizophrenia, not a positive (psychotic) symptom. Avolition is an absence of motivation for goal-oriented behaviors. The term *positive* refers not to something of positive valuation but rather to something that is present and existing, as opposed to a deficit symptom such as the negative symptoms of schizophrenia. The other symptom types listed are considered psychotic.

**19—Key Features That Define the Psychotic Disorders / Negative Symptoms (p. 88)**

20. What is the most common type of delusion?

   A. Somatic delusion of distorted body appearance.
   B. Grandiose delusion.
   C. Thought insertion.
   D. Persecutory delusion.
   E. Former life regression.

**Correct Answer: D. Persecutory delusion.**

**Explanation:** Persecutory delusions are the most common form. This may be because such delusions are associated with a dysregulation of existing self-protective and/or social-psychological functionalities, but the reason that these are the most commonly encountered delusion is not yet well understood.

**20—Key Features That Define the Psychotic Disorders / Delusions (p. 87)**

21. Label each of the following beliefs as a bizarre delusion, a nonbizarre delusion, or a nondelusion.

   A. A 25-year-old law student believes he has uncovered the truth about JFK's assassination and that CIA agents have been dispatched to follow him and monitor his Internet communications.
   B. A 45-year-old homeless man presents to the psychiatric emergency room complaining of a skin rash. Upon removal of his clothes, it is seen that most of his body is wrapped in aluminum foil. The man explains that he is protecting himself from the electromagnetic ray guns that are constantly targeting him.
   C. A 47-year-old unemployed plumber believes he has been elected to the House of Representatives. When the Capitol police evict him and bring him to the emergency department, he says that they are Tea Party activists who are merely impersonating police officers.

D. A 35-year-old high school physics teacher presents to your office with insomnia and tells you that he has discovered and memorized the formula for cold fusion energy, only to have the formula removed from his memory by telepathic aliens.

E. An 18-year-old recent immigrant from Eastern Europe believes that wearing certain colors will ward off the "evil eye" and prevent catastrophes that would otherwise occur.

**Correct Answer: A, nonbizarre delusion; B, bizarre delusion; C, nonbizarre delusion; D, bizarre delusion; E, nondelusion.**

**Explanation:** Delusions are deemed bizarre if they are clearly implausible and not understandable to same-culture peers and do not derive from ordinary life experiences. Thus, although it is probably untrue that the law student is being followed and that the plumber has been elected to Congress, these things *could* conceivably happen. By contrast, thought removal and external control by telepathically empowered aliens or electromagnetic ray guns is not in the realm of possibility by shared social consensus. The belief that use of colors or amulets will ward off bad events is an accepted part of many cultural belief systems and so is not classifiable as a delusion, even if it seems implausible to individuals from more secular backgrounds.

21—Key Features That Define the Psychotic Disorders / Delusions (p. 87); Schizophrenia / Culture-Related Diagnostic Issues (p. 103)

22. Which of the following presentations would *not* be classified as disorganized behavior for the purpose of diagnosing schizophrenia spectrum and other psychotic disorders?

A. Masturbating in public.
B. Wearing slacks on one's head.
C. Responding verbally to auditory hallucinations in a conversational mode.
D. Crouching on all fours and barking.
E. Turning to face 180 degrees away from the interviewer when answering questions.

**Correct Answer: C. Responding verbally to auditory hallucinations in a conversational mode.**

**Explanation:** Disorganized behavior including catatonic motor behavior is one of four categories of psychotic symptoms used to diagnose schizophrenia spectrum and other psychotic disorders. To fulfill diagnostic criteria, the behavior must be grossly disorganized or inappropriate. Masturbating in public is behavior that shows obliviousness to the environment and unconcern for the usual social norms of modesty and privacy. Wearing clothing in odd ways without justification is a disorganized form of behavior. Both barking like a dog and turning away in a bizarre fashion while conducting a conversation (if not induced by an expression of anger or other reasonable explanation) are grossly inappropriate behaviors. However, responding verbally to auditory hallucination is not in itself a disorganized behavior. Given the belief in the actuality of communication in an auditory hallucination, talking back is contingently a logical and goal-oriented behavior. Thus, this would count as one psychotic symptom (hallucination) but not as two symptoms (hallucination and grossly disorganized behavior).

**22—Key Features That Define the Psychotic Disorders / Grossly Disorganized or Abnormal Motor Behavior (Including Catatonia) (p. 88)**

23. Which of the following statements about catatonic motor behaviors is *false?*

    A. Catatonic motor behavior is a type of grossly disorganized behavior that has historically been associated with schizophrenia spectrum and other psychotic disorders.
    B. Catatonic motor behaviors may occur in many mental disorders (such as mood disorders) and in other medical conditions.
    C. A behavior is considered catatonic only if it involves motoric slowing or rigidity, such as mutism, posturing, or waxy flexibility.
    D. Catatonia can be diagnosed independently of another psychiatric disorder.
    E. Catatonic behaviors involve markedly reduced reactivity to the environment.

    **Correct Answer: C. A behavior is considered catatonic only if it involves motoric slowing or rigidity, such as mutism, posturing, or waxy flexibility.**

    **Explanation:** *Catatonic behavior* is a marked decrease in reactivity to the environment. This ranges from resistance to instructions (negativism); to maintaining a rigid, inappropriate or bizarre posture; to a complete lack of verbal and motor responses (mutism and stupor). It can also include purposeless and excessive motor activity without obvious cause (catatonic excitement). Other features are repeated stereotyped movements, staring, grimacing, mutism, and the echoing of speech. Although catatonia has historically been associated with schizophrenia, catatonic symptoms are nonspecific and may occur in other mental disorders (e.g., bipolar or depressive disorders with catatonia) and in medical conditions (catatonic disorder due to another medical condition).

    **23—Key Features That Define the Psychotic Disorders / Grossly Disorganized or Abnormal Motor Behavior (Including Catatonia) (p. 88); Catatonia (pp. 119–121)**

24. Which of the following statements about negative symptoms of schizophrenia is *false?*

    A. Negative symptoms are easily distinguished from medication side effects such as sedation.
    B. Negative symptoms include diminished emotional expression.

C. Negative symptoms can be difficult to distinguish from medication side effects such as sedation.
D. Negative symptoms include reduced peer or social interaction.
E. Negative symptoms include decreased motivation for goal-directed activities.

**Correct Answer: A. Negative symptoms are easily distinguished from medication side effects such as sedation.**

**Explanation:** Negative symptoms of schizophrenia refer to the deficit aspects of the illness, in contrast to the "positive" symptoms (in the sense of being notable by their presence, not in the sense of being desirable). Positive symptoms include active hallucinations, delusions, disorganized behaviors, and disorganized thinking. Side effects of medication such as sedation and bradykinesia may mimic negative symptoms and be wrongly evaluated as primary negative symptomatology. The primary negative symptoms include diminished emotional expression, reduced interaction with others, and decreased motivation for goal-directed activities.

**24—Key Features That Define the Psychotic Disorders / Negative Symptoms (p. 88)**

25. Which of the following statements correctly describes a way in which schizoaffective disorder may be differentiated from bipolar disorder?

A. Schizoaffective disorder involves only depressive episodes, never manic or hypomanic episodes.
B. In bipolar disorder, psychotic symptoms do not last longer than 1 month.
C. In bipolar disorder, psychotic symptoms are always cotemporal with mood symptoms.
D. Schizoaffective disorder never includes full-blown episodes of major depression.
E. In bipolar disorder, psychotic symptoms are always mood congruent.

**Correct Answer: C. In bipolar disorder, psychotic symptoms are always cotemporal with mood symptoms.**

**Explanation:** Distinguishing schizoaffective disorder from depressive and bipolar disorders with psychotic features is often difficult. Schizoaffective disorder can be distinguished from a depressive or bipolar disorder with psychotic features by the presence of prominent delusions and/or hallucinations for at least 2 weeks in the absence of a major mood episode. In contrast, in depressive or bipolar disorders with psychotic features, the psychotic features primarily occur during the mood episode(s).

**25—Schizoaffective Disorder / Differential Diagnosis (pp. 109–110)**

26. Which of the following symptom combinations, if present for 1 month, would meet Criterion A for schizophrenia?

    A. Prominent auditory and visual hallucinations.
    B. Grossly disorganized behavior and avolition.
    C. Disorganized speech and diminished emotional expression.
    D. Paranoid and grandiose delusions.
    E. Avolition and diminished emotional expression.

    **Correct Answer: C. Disorganized speech and diminished emotional expression.**

    **Explanation:** To meet DSM-5 Criterion A, two (or more) of the following symptoms must be present for a significant portion of time during a 1-month period (or less if successfully treated): 1) delusions, 2) hallucinations, 3) disorganized speech (e.g., frequent derailment or incoherence), 4) grossly disorganized or catatonic behavior, 5) negative symptoms (i.e., diminished emotional expression or avolition). At least one of the two symptoms must be the clear presence of delusions (A1), hallucinations (A2), or disorganized speech (A3). Thus, two forms of hallucinations or two types of delusions alone in the absence of other symptoms would be insufficient to meet Criterion A. The combination of grossly disorganized behavior (although considered a psychotic symptom) with negative symptoms is also insufficient to meet Criterion A.

    26—Schizophrenia / diagnostic criteria (pp. 99–100)

27. Which of the following statements about violent or suicidal behavior in schizophrenia is *false?*

    A. About 5%–6% of individuals with schizophrenia die by suicide.
    B. Persons with schizophrenia frequently assault strangers in a random fashion.
    C. Compared with the general population, persons with schizophrenia are more frequently victims of violence.
    D. Command hallucinations to harm oneself sometimes precede suicidal behaviors.
    E. Youth, male gender, and substance abuse are factors that increase the risk for suicide among persons with schizophrenia.

    **Correct Answer: B. Persons with schizophrenia frequently assault strangers in a random fashion.**

    **Explanation:** Hostility and aggression can be associated with schizophrenia, although spontaneous or random assault is uncommon. Aggression is more frequent for younger males and for individuals with a past history of violence, nonadherence to treatment, substance abuse, and impulsivity. It should be noted that the vast majority of persons with schizophrenia are not aggressive and are more frequently victimized than are individuals in the general population.

Approximately 5%–6% of individuals with schizophrenia die by suicide, about 20% attempt suicide on one or more occasions, and many more have significant suicidal ideation. Suicidal behavior is sometimes in response to command hallucinations to harm oneself or others. Suicide risk remains high over the whole life span for males and females, although it may be especially high for younger males with comorbid substance use. Other risk factors include having depressive symptoms or feelings of hopelessness and being unemployed, and the risk is higher, also, in the period after a psychotic episode or hospital discharge.

27—Schizophrenia / Associated Features Supporting Diagnosis (pp. 101–102); Suicide Risk (p. 104)

28. Which of the following statements about childhood-onset schizophrenia is *true?*

A. Childhood-onset schizophrenia tends to resemble poor-outcome adult schizophrenia, with gradual onset and prominent negative symptoms.
B. Disorganized speech patterns in childhood are usually indicative of schizophrenia.
C. Because of the childhood capacity for imagination, delusions and hallucinations in childhood-onset schizophrenia are more elaborate than those in adult-onset schizophrenia.
D. In a child presenting with disorganized behavior, schizophrenia should be ruled out before other childhood diagnoses are considered.
E. Visual hallucinations are extremely rare in childhood-onset schizophrenia.

**Correct Answer: A. Childhood-onset schizophrenia tends to resemble poor-outcome adult schizophrenia, with gradual onset and prominent negative symptoms.**

**Explanation:** The essential features of schizophrenia are the same in childhood, but it is more difficult to make the diagnosis. In children, delusions and hallucinations may be less elaborate than in adults, and visual hallucinations are more common and should be distinguished from normal fantasy play. Disorganized speech occurs in many disorders with childhood onset (e.g., autism spectrum disorder), as does disorganized behavior (e.g., attention-deficit/hyperactivity disorder). These symptoms should not be attributed to schizophrenia without due consideration of the more common disorders of childhood. Childhood-onset cases tend to resemble poor-outcome adult cases, with gradual onset and prominent negative symptoms. Children who later receive the diagnosis of schizophrenia are more likely to have experienced nonspecific emotional-behavioral disturbances and psychopathology, intellectual and language alterations, and subtle motor delays.

28—Schizophrenia / Development and Course (pp. 102–103)

29. Which of the following statements about gender differences in schizophrenia is *true?*

   A. Women with schizophrenia tend to have fewer psychotic symptoms than do men over the course of the illness.
   B. A first onset of schizophrenia after age 40 is more likely in women than in men.
   C. Psychotic symptoms in women tend to burn out with age to a greater extent than they do in men.
   D. Negative symptoms and affective flattening are more frequently observed in women with schizophrenia than in men with the disorder.
   E. The overall incidence of schizophrenia is higher in women than it is in men.

   **Correct Answer: B. A first onset of schizophrenia after age 40 is more likely in women than in men.**

   **Explanation:** The lifetime prevalence of schizophrenia appears to be approximately 0.3%–0.7%, although there is reported variation by race/ethnicity, across countries, and by geographic origin for immigrants and children of immigrants. The sex ratio differs across samples and populations: for example, an emphasis on negative symptoms and longer duration of disorder (associated with poorer outcome) shows higher incidence rates for males, whereas definitions allowing for the inclusion of more mood symptoms and brief presentations (associated with better outcome) show equivalent risks for both sexes.
   A number of features distinguish the clinical expression of schizophrenia in females and males. The general incidence of schizophrenia tends to be slightly lower in females, particularly among treated cases. The age at onset is later in females, with a second mid-life peak. Symptoms tend to be more affect-laden among females, and there are more psychotic symptoms, as well as a greater propensity for psychotic symptoms to worsen in later life. Other symptom differences include less frequent negative symptoms and disorganization. Finally, social functioning tends to remain better preserved in females. There are, however, frequent exceptions to these general caveats.

   **29—Schizophrenia / Prevalence (p. 102); Gender-Related Diagnostic Issues (pp. 103–104)**

30. A 19-year-old female college student is brought to the emergency department by her family over her objections. Three months ago, she suddenly started feeling "odd," and she came home from college because she could not concentrate. Two weeks after she came home, she began hearing voices telling her that she is "a sinner" and must repent. Although never a religious person, she now believes she must repent, but she does not know how, and feels confused. She is managing her activities of daily living despite the ongoing auditory hallucinations and delusions, and she is affectively reactive on examination. Which diagnosis best fits this presentation?

   A. Schizophreniform disorder, with good prognostic features, provisional.
   B. Schizophreniform disorder, without good prognostic features, provisional.

    C. Schizophreniform disorder, with good prognostic features.

    D. Schizophreniform disorder, without good prognostic features.

    E. Unspecified schizophrenia spectrum and other psychotic disorder.

**Correct Answer: A. Schizophreniform disorder, with good prognostic features, provisional.**

**Explanation:** Schizophreniform disorder is diagnosed under two conditions: 1) when an episode of illness lasts between 1 and 6 months and the individual has already recovered, and 2) when an individual is symptomatic for less than the 6 months' duration required for the diagnosis of schizophrenia but has not yet recovered (as in this vignette). One then adds the qualifier "provisional," because it is uncertain whether the individual will recover from the disturbance within the 6-month period. If the disturbance persists beyond 6 months, the diagnosis should be changed to schizophrenia. In either case, schizophreniform disorder takes the specifier "with good prognostic features" if at least two of the following features are present: 1) onset of prominent psychotic symptoms within 4 weeks of the first noticeable change in usual behavior or functioning; 2) confusion or perplexity; 3) good premorbid social and occupational functioning; and 4) absence of blunted or flat affect. This vignette demonstrates all four of these features. Because we have enough information to make the diagnosis of schizophreniform disorder, unspecified schizophrenia spectrum and other psychotic disorder would be incorrectly applied.

    30—Schizophreniform Disorder / diagnostic criteria (pp. 96–97); Diagnostic Features
        (pp. 97–98)

31. A 24-year-old male college student is brought to the emergency department by the college health service team. A few weeks ago he was involved in a car accident in which one of his friends was critically injured and died in his arms. The man has not come out of his room or showered for the last 2 weeks. He has eaten only minimally, claimed that aliens have targeted him for abduction, and asserted that he could hear their radio transmissions. Nothing seems to convince him that this abduction will not happen or that the transmissions are not real. Which of the following diagnoses (and justifications) is most appropriate for this man?

    A. Brief psychotic disorder with a marked stressor, because the symptoms began after the tragic car accident.

    B. Brief psychotic disorder without a marked stressor, because the content of the psychosis is unrelated to the accident.

    C. Unspecified schizophrenia spectrum and other psychotic disorder, because more information is needed.

    D. Schizophreniform disorder, because there are psychotic symptoms but not yet a full-blown schizophrenia picture.

    E. Delusional disorder, because the central symptom is a delusion of persecution.

**Correct Answer: C. Unspecified schizophrenia spectrum and other psychotic disorder, because more information is needed.**

**Explanation:** The diagnosis of *brief psychotic disorder* requires that there be psychotic symptoms lasting more than 1 day but less than 1 month and that the patient has shown a full recovery. In this vignette, we do not know how long the symptoms will last or whether the patient will fully recover. If the patient's symptoms remit in less than 1 month and he shows full recovery, one could diagnose *brief psychotic disorder with a marked stressor*. There is no requirement that the content of the psychotic symptoms match the events that constitute the stressor, as long as the temporal sequence holds. The diagnosis of *delusional disorder* requires 1 month of symptoms and does not usually involve bizarre delusions, nor does it involve the functional deficits seen here. *Schizophreniform disorder* requires 1 month of symptoms. If these symptoms continue for a month and functional deficits persist, the diagnosis could be schizophreniform disorder, and possibly progress to schizophrenia after 6 months. We do not yet know the future trajectory of these psychotic symptoms and therefore can justify only the diagnosis of unspecified schizophrenia spectrum and other psychotic disorder. The unspecified schizophrenia spectrum and other psychotic disorder category is used in situations in which the clinician chooses not to specify the reason that the criteria are not met for a specific schizophrenia spectrum and other psychotic disorder, and includes presentations in which there is insufficient information to make a more specific diagnosis (e.g., in emergency room settings).

31—Unspecified Schizophrenia Spectrum and Other Psychotic Disorder (p. 122)